Comments on Cancer information at your fingertips *from readers*

'I think it is an excellent book and will be of enormous value to anyone who is diagnosed with cancer and, equally important, their close family members. The authors are to be congratulated on making a valuable contribution to the continuing campaign to overcome and, hopefully, prevent cancer.'

Mike Shaw, Tunbridge Wells

'Thank you very much for a helpful book, to which I shall constantly turn and pass on to others. It is just the book I was looking for, as I know nothing about cancer from a medical point of view.'

Rev Ronald Monk, Bacup, Lincs

'I thoroughly recommend this book to all people who are anxious about either having cancer, suspecting they may have cancer, or have a dear friend or relation where cancer has been diagnosed. It will dispel many rumours, doubts and fears.

This reference book is very easily understood and does not contain what I would consider oblique medical jargon. The basic approach is most welcome to the ordinary, everyday person.

May you derive comfort and determination from it.'

Roy Castle, entertainer and TV personality

'The book contains a lot of very valuable information, and is extremely useful as a reference guide.'

Bob Champion, leading National Hunt jockey

'I have read **Cancer information at your fingertips** more than once and I think it is an excellent book for people with cancer and their families. It answered just about every question I had in a clear and concise fashion.'

Nicki Hutchinson, Chichester

'This isn't just a book for those who have cancer – it's for their relatives and carers as well. As the closest relative of a sufferer, I often felt as if I couldn't ask his consultant the questions which I needed answering – I was concerned I'd be wasting his time and that I'd be asking questions he couldn't be able to answer or wouldn't want to answer or had answered already.'

Jo Langford, London

Reviews of **Cancer information at your fingertips**

'Occasionally I come across a book that I wish that I had written, and this is one. Written in question and answer format and divided into broad category chapters, it is simple and yet not condescending in its approach!

I have no hesitation in recommending this book to anyone needing more information about cancer. A truly useful reference book.'

Kay Wright, Cancer Nursing Society Newsletter

'People with cancer need honest information if they are to understand their condition and make rational choices about treatment. The authors of this manual ... have combined their considerable experience and knowledge to produce a useful source of information for patients with cancer and their families.

I shall recommend this book to patients with cancer who want to learn more about their condition.'

David Jeffrey, European Journal of Cancer Care

'The book is understandable and easy to read, written by two experts in the field of communicating with patients ... It is also an extremely valuable book for nononcology health professionals to have by (or under) their desk to help them answer difficult questions!'

Professor B. W. Hancock, Hospital Update

'This is definitely a book to recommend to our patients and their relatives, but health professionals could also glean much useful information.'

Caroline Richens, Nursing Standard

'Cancer patients often have many questions about their illness, but busy doctors don't always have time to give all the answers. This is an excellent guide for anyone facing cancer, from the early days when the disease is still being diagnosed right through to the completion of treatment and getting back to normal life.'

Alison Wick, Woman magazine

'It's the kind of book that makes you think 'Why didn't someone do this ages ago?' **Cancer information at your fingertips** is an excellent guide for those cancer sufferers, their families and friends who want to be aware of what is happening, and hopefully how they can take some control over it.'

Centrepiece – the Bristol Cancer Help Centre Newsletter

Cancer information at your fingertips

THE COMPREHENSIVE CANCER REFERENCE BOOK FOR THE YEAR 2000

Val Speechley, MA, RGN, RCNT, Oncology Nursing Certificate
Senior nurse, Patient information and education, The Royal Marsden Hospital, London and Surrey

Maxine Rosenfield DCRT, Dip.Couns.
Helpline trainer and consultant, Broadcasting Support Services; former Head of CancerLink Information Service

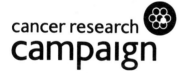
cancer research
campaign

THE BRITISH SCHOOL OF OSTEOPATHY
1-4 SUFFOLK ST., LONDON. SW1Y 4HG
TEL. 01 - 930 9254-8

A percentage of the revenue from sales of this book will go directly to the Cancer Research Campaign
(Registered Charity No. 225838)

CLASS PUBLISHING · LONDON

Printing history
First published 1992
Reprinted with corrections 1992
Second edition 1996

The authors and publishers welcome feedback from the users of this book.
Please contact the publishers.

**Class Publishing (London) Ltd, 7 Melrose Terrace, London W6 7RL, UK
Telephone: 0171 371 2119
Fax: 0171 371 2878 [International +44171]**

A CIP catalogue record for this book is available from the British Library

ISBN 1 872362 56 7

Designed by Wendy Bann

Edited and indexed by Susan Bosanko

Production by Landmark Production Consultants Ltd, Princes Risborough

Typesetting by DP Photosetting, Aylesbury, Bucks

Printed by Butler and Tanner Ltd, Frome

Contents

Foreword

by Professor J. Gordon McVie

Scientific Director, Cancer Research Campaign

Cancer patients are beset by doubts. And doubts are formulated into questions. And questions need answers. I cannot recall a patient nor relative nor friend who didn't seek the reassurance which comes from authoritative answers to their troubled questions. And this book provides them. Roy Castle read the first edition of this book shortly before his tragic death from lung cancer. He was not always complimentary about the caring professions' communication skills, language or techniques, but he strongly endorsed this book. So do I.

Gordon McVie

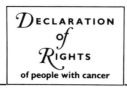

DECLARATION of RIGHTS
of people with cancer

These rights have been identified by people with cancer as being essential to their wellbeing. They are not all legal rights.

I have the right:

1. ... to equal concern and attention whatever my gender, race, class, culture, religious belief, age, sexuality, lifestyle or degree of able-bodiedness.

2. ... to be considered with respect and dignity, and to have my physical, emotional, spiritual, social and psychological needs taken seriously and responded to throughout my life, whatever my prognosis.

3. ... to know I have cancer, to be told in a sensitive manner and to share in all decision-making about my treatment and care in honest and informative discussions with relevant specialists and other health professionals.

4. ... to be informed fully about treatment options and to have explained to me the benefits, side effects and risks of any treatment.

5. ... to be asked for my informed consent before I am entered into any clinical trial.

6. ... to a second opinion, to refuse treatment or to use complementary therapies without prejudice to continued medical support.

7. ... to have any special welfare needs acknowledged and benefit claims responded to promptly.

8. ... to be employed, promoted or accepted on return to work according to my abilities and experience and not according to assumptions made about my disease and its progression.

9. ... to easy access to information about local and national services, cancer support and self help groups and practitioners that may be useful in meeting my needs.

10. ... to receive support and information to help me understand and come to terms with my disease, and to receive similar support for my family and friends.

Reproduced by kind permission of CancerLink.

Introduction

This book consists of a series of questions and answers that provide information about cancer, the treatment options available and ways of living with – and after – treatment for cancer. It is intended to be used by people who have cancer and their friends and relatives.

The contents are based on the most commonly asked questions about cancer, drawn from various sources including the authors' personal experience. While it attempts to be comprehensive and to touch on all aspects of the disease, we are conscious that there are omissions. To include every possible fact or facet would require an encyclopaedia!

Similarly the answers given will not be relevant to every individual in every situation. It is essential that people with cancer ask questions of their doctors, nurses and other health care professionals. It is equally important that they gain easy, unprejudiced access to the voluntary and supportive services which exist. Hopefully the result will be a better understanding of their experiences and of how to live a full life with, and after, cancer.

This book aims to give you accurate information to enable you to exercise some or all of the rights listed opposite, if you so wish.

The chapters are arranged to answer questions about cancer facts, how a cancer diagnosis is made, the hospital treatments which may be offered, their possible side effects, complementary therapies which may be used and the ways in which cancer can affect your lifestyle.

You may decide to read the book from cover to cover, but it has been written so that you can choose the parts in which you are most interested. For this reason, some of the information is repeated in more than one chapter, but we think it is better to repeat information at all the points where it might be needed than to ask you to keep moving from one place in the book to another.

We would like to know if there are important questions we have not covered (which we may be able to incorporate in a later edition) and we would also welcome any other comments you may have on this book. Please write to us c/o Class Publishing, 7 Melrose Terrace, London W6 7RL, UK.

We would like to thank David Proudfoot, who patiently typed and revised the manuscript often under considerable pressure. He hardly ever lost his temper!

1
What is cancer?

Introduction

Cancer is a single word which is used to describe about 200 different diseases affecting organs or systems throughout our bodies. Each form of cancer is unique in terms of its development, possible causes and behaviour. The language used to describe cancer is also complicated because of all the different types of cancer and how they are subdivided. Some common terms are explained here and advice is offered about how to reduce your risk of developing cancer.

What is cancer?

Cancer is a disease of cells. These are the smallest building blocks in our bodies, invisible to the naked eye. Groups of cells form the tissues and organs of the body (such as the brain, liver, kidneys or lungs): each of these has a very specific function.

Cells normally reproduce themselves by dividing in a regular, orderly fashion so that growth and repair of the body tissues can take place. If this normal function is disrupted, there may be an uncontrolled growth of cells causing a swelling or **tumour**. Tumours may be benign or malignant.

Benign tumours remain contained within a localised area and once treated, often by an operation, do not usually cause any further problems. A wart is an example of a benign tumour.

Cancers or **malignant** tumours have two special features: they can spread to or infiltrate nearby organs or tissues, and

1

cancer cells can break off the original tumour and may be carried in the bloodstream to distant sites in the body where they may form new tumours called **metastases** or **secondaries**. Cancer cells may also be carried in the lymphatic system, which normally helps the body to fight infection. The lymphatic system also takes fluid from different parts of the body and returns it to the bloodstream.

It is because cancer cells can spread to vital organs (such as the lungs or liver) and affect their normal function that cancer anywhere in the body is a potentially life-threatening disease.

The doctor told me I have a neoplasm. What's the difference between this and a tumour?

Tumour means swelling, neoplasm means new growth and doctors may also refer to lesions or ulcers. All these terms can be used to describe either a benign condition or a malignant one, so the important question to ask is 'Have I got cancer?'.

Leukaemia is a form of cancer, isn't it? Why are there are no lumps?

Malignant changes occur when cells go out of control and prevent the normal function of an organ or system. This may take the form of a solid tumour which affects the mechanics of an organ. For example, a lung cancer can prevent the lungs expanding properly causing breathing difficulties, or a bowel cancer can create a blockage. Alternatively the rogue cells may multiply rapidly and replace the normal cells without forming solid 'lumps'. This is what happens in leukaemia.

Leukaemia is cancer of the white blood cells which are formed in the bone marrow. The healthy blood cells, whose function is to carry oxygen around the body, fight infection and help the blood to clot, are pushed out by the abnormal cells. The reduced numbers of normal cells are unable to function properly and the person becomes anaemic and vulnerable to infection and haemorrhage.

Why doesn't the body fight back?

The body does fight back against cancer cells using the white blood cells and the lymphatic system. It is probable that for every cancer that develops to the extent that it affects the body there have been many others which have been destroyed in the very early stages. However, the cancer cells may simply overwhelm the body's defence systems and continue to grow. Even if this happens cancer spread may be stopped or slowed down by these same defence systems and it may be possible to remove all the cancer with an operation.

Doctors are often confident that they have removed all the cancer and yet it comes back years later. Why does this happen?

Cancers usually take many years to grow to the size, or number of cells, which causes a sign or symptom which is troublesome and leads someone to contact their doctor. During this period there is plenty of time for cells to break off the original tumour and spread to other parts of the body. When the doctor examines the person and asks for tests to be done these new tumours may be so small as to go undetected. Even if all the original cancer appears to have been removed, or there is no evidence of disease after treatment, the secondary tumours may already be growing at other sites. They may stay 'silent' for months or years, just as the original cancer did, until the cells reach sufficient numbers to cause a new symptom. It only requires one cancer cell to be left undetected or untreated for a recurrence of the disease to occur in the future.

I thought cancer only occurred in old people but recently a friend of my son's was told he had cancer. How did this happen?

Cancer is mainly a disease of older people, with seven out of 10 of all new cases occurring in people who are over 60 years old. However, malignant changes in cells can occur at any age and certain cancers develop more frequently in children and young people or are specific to these age groups.

If there are lots of different cancers which can develop at various times in our lives how do doctors decide what type of cancer someone has?

Cancers are grouped or **classified** according to the type of cell from which they develop. Some examples are **carcinomas**, which arise from the epithelium (lining) of an organ or system, and **sarcomas**, which occur because of changes in the supportive tissues of the body (such as muscle and bone).

Within these general classifications there are further subdivisions, such as **adeno**carcinomas if the original cell is from a gland lining an organ, and **osteo**sarcomas if the supporting tissue is a bone.

There are also less common malignancies of the blood-forming cells, such as **leukaemia** (white blood cells), **myeloma** (plasma cells), and **lymphoma** (the lymphatic system). In the nervous system changes in supportive cells are called **gliomas**, while those affecting the immature nerve cells are called **neuroblastomas**. Cancers of the reproductive cells are termed **seminomas** or **teratomas**, the latter occurring in both young men and women.

All these divisions and sub-divisions are made even more complex because the malignant cells may be similar to normal cells or they may bear little resemblance to them. This similarity, or lack of it, is called **differentiation**.

When doctors suspect that someone has a cancerous tumour, or a malignant disease like leukaemia, they will ask for a sample of the cells to be sent to a **cytologist**, who will examine them under a microscope and identify which type of cancer is present.

What are the most common types of cancer?

The most common types of cancer are carcinomas. In the United Kingdom the organs most frequently affected by these are the lung, breast, skin, colon and rectum (bowel), prostate, stomach, bladder, ovary and cervix. The incidence of cancer varies from country to country throughout the world and sometimes from city to countryside and region to region.

There seems to be more written about cancer in newspapers and magazines now, and more programmes on television. Is cancer a new disease?

No, cancer has existed for thousands of years. Records of cases of cancer and how it was treated have been found in ancient Egyptian mummies and in the records of Greek civilisation.

Is cancer becoming more common?

It is difficult to give a simple yes or no answer to this question. The **incidence** of cancer, that is the number of new cases each year for every million people in the population, varies from country to country, and from one type of cancer to another. Many things affect the figures, for example average life expectancy, how accurately records are kept, and people's personal habits such as smoking and sunbathing. In this country, people are living longer and the records of how many people develop cancer are now very accurate, so when we compare figures it appears that there are more cases of cancer than there used to be. However, while certain types of cancer, such as skin cancer, are now seen more often in the UK, the incidence of others, such as stomach cancer, is falling. It is a very complicated topic!

If cancer isn't a new disease and it isn't that much more common now, why do we hear more about it?

There are lots of reasons why cancer has become a more prominent health issue. Improvements in public health and treatments or cures for other serious illnesses (such as TB) which led to premature death mean that people are living longer. The risk of developing the most common cancers increases with age so living longer means that more people will have cancer, as most new cases occur in people who are over 60 years old. In addition, people are more willing to talk openly about cancer now, so we hear about individuals or celebrities who have survived the disease.

Is cancer the main cause of death in this country?

No, twice as many people die of cardiovascular disease (heart attacks and problems with the circulation of the blood). Cancer is second in line but people tend to be more scared of developing it. They think they will always die, often quickly, and that inevitably this will be painful and unpleasant in some way. This is not true.

What is my chance of getting cancer?

One in three people will develop cancer at some time during their life but this will depend to some extent on their personal habits, their job and the environment.

If I do get cancer I'll probably die from it, won't I?

No, one in three of the people who develop cancer are cured of their disease. Many more live for years without problems directly associated with their cancer. They may eventually die of the cancer but a diagnosis of cancer is not an automatic sentence of death.

What causes cancer?

Every cell in the body contains a set of instructions (its genetic material) which control the way it grows and behaves. Cancer happens when changes take place in this genetic material so that the cells no longer behave normally and instead grow in an uncontrolled way. There are many reasons why this may happen. Cancer is not one disease, therefore the search is not for a single cause. Scientists know that the process of malignant (cancerous) change is very complicated and this is why doctors often refer to **predisposing factors**, that is things which are common to people who develop a particular type of cancer. Research has shown a direct link between some personal habits and cancer, for example between smoking and lung cancer. It is also known that exposure to radiation can cause cancer. Marie Curie, who discovered radioactivity, died of cancer. Some substances, for example chemicals like vinyl chloride, arsenic and certain dyes, are known to be **carcinogens** (cancer-causing agents). Even so, when we consider an individual person none of these factors may be present and the reason why a cancer has developed remains a mystery.

Some cancers seem to run in families. Can you inherit cancer?

It is very rare that a cancer is passed from generation to generation like the colour of one's eyes or hair. One example of this is an extremely rare eye tumour called **retinoblastoma**, which affects about 40 children a year in the UK. However, some families do seem to have a tendency to develop a particular type of cancer, for example cancers of the breast, bowel or ovary, or they may have other inherited conditions which are known to be pre-cancerous. An example of such a condition is **polyposis coli**, in which polyps (small growths) develop in the colon (large bowel).

Why do more cases of cancer occur in some families?

That is difficult to say, especially if members of the family develop different types of cancer. It may be coincidence or something to do with the family's lifestyle. There may be an inherited risk of developing cancer passed on through the genes, which determine family characteristics. A great deal of research is being carried out at the moment to discover if a fault in a particular gene is responsible for this increased risk.

If a gene was found that showed a person had an increased risk of developing cancer, could cancer be prevented?

It might be possible one day to prevent cancer in this way but it will be a few years before we know for sure. There are thousands of genes to examine, and faults in different genes may be responsible for the development of different cancers. So far scientists have discovered two types of genes which control cell growth. One type is called an **oncogene** (onco = tumour), which encourages cells to grow; the other is called a **tumour suppressor gene**, which stops cells growing. Research into identifying cancer genes is continuing. Eventually doctors may be able to change genes in some way (for example by reforming or repairing them or switching them off) to reduce a person's risk of getting cancer, but at present we have to look to what we already know to prevent the disease.

What can I do to reduce my risk of getting cancer?

Everyone can do certain things to reduce the likelihood of getting cancer. We probably all carry genes such as those described in the previous question but something external is needed to 'trigger' the uncontrolled division of cells which leads to formation of a cancer, or to stop the tumour suppressor genes from working normally to prevent a cancer developing. When we think about reducing the risk of cancer we need to look at two main areas: our lifestyle (personal habits), and our occupation or job.

Some things we can't control - we all get older and our immune system (bodily defence system) does not work so efficiently; we can't influence our normal hormone levels, which might affect how our cells behave; and we can't easily change our environment and where we live, which sometimes seems to have a bearing on what type of cancer we may develop (for example, cancer of the ovary appears to be more common in rural communities - the reason is unknown).

All of the aspects of our lives discussed in the next few questions are equally important for people who are living with cancer.

Does smoking cause cancer?

Yes. There is now no doubt that smoking causes cancer as well as many other serious health problems. Between 80-90% of all cases of lung cancer are associated with smoking and cancer of the larynx (voice box), oesophagus (gullet), bladder and pancreas are all seen more frequently in smokers. Cigarettes are the main culprit but pipe and cigar smokers also run an increased risk of mouth and throat cancer. Women have an increased risk of cancer of the cervix.

The risk of developing cancer is increased by the amount of tobacco you smoke and how long you have been smoking. So if you don't smoke, don't start and if you do, try to reduce your consumption or, best of all, stop altogether. As soon as you stop your risk of developing cancer starts to fall and in 15 years that risk will be the same as if you had never smoked.

Is it safe to chew tobacco?

No. Chewing tobacco or tobacco packets (skol bandits) may cause cancer of the mouth. Skol bandits are illegal in the UK.

Does my risk of lung cancer rise if I live with a smoker but don't smoke myself?

Yes. The dangers of what is called passive smoking are now well known. Your risk of getting lung cancer could be 10-30% higher.

How do I stop smoking?

There is lots of help available nowadays to assist people to give up smoking. Your family doctor or local health education unit should be able to offer advice and support.

What about the side effects of giving up smoking?

Lots of people worry about the side effects, such as putting on weight or not being able to relax. Side effects are only temporary - you can usually lose any extra pounds by being careful about what you eat, or if you are irritable or tense there are many ways to relax, such as listening to special cassettes. The benefits to your social life, to the amount of money in your pocket and to your health will far outweigh any difficulties you have at first.

Does drinking alcohol cause cancer?

Certain types of cancer are more common in heavy drinkers. These include cancers of the mouth, throat, oesophagus (gullet) and liver. It appears that the combination of heavy drinking and heavy smoking is most damaging.

This does not mean that you have to give up alcohol altogether. The golden rule is to drink in moderation. Your local health education unit or your doctor will be able to give you advice on what is sensible drinking. The recommended amount is a maximum of 21 units each week for men and 14 units each week for women (one unit of alcohol equals half a pint of beer or cider, one glass of wine or a single measure of spirits).

There's a saying 'you are what you eat'. Can changing my diet reduce my risk of getting cancer?

There is some evidence that changing your diet may affect your chances of developing cancer. For example, we do know that eating plenty of fruit and vegetables reduces the risk of cancer of the digestive and respiratory systems. It is thought that about one-third of cancers may be linked to poor diet.

Researchers have looked at the incidence of certain cancers in countries throughout the world and have found that patterns can be seen. For example, breast cancer is more common in countries where people eat a diet which contains large amounts of fat and bowel cancer is less common when people eat plenty of fibre (roughage). However, if you look at one person with either of these cancers it may not be possible to identify anything in their diet which could have caused the cancer.

What about watching my weight?

There are many good reasons for keeping your weight within the normal range for your height, not least that it will reduce your risk of developing heart disease. There is some evidence that cancer of the uterus (womb) occurs more often in women who are obese (overweight).

I've heard that if you take lots of vitamins it will protect against cancer. Is this true?

Some studies suggest that vitamins A, E and C, and a substance called beta-carotene may offer protection against cancer. Research is continuing to discover if a link can be proved. If you eat a well balanced, healthy diet you should get enough of these vitamins naturally and not need to take vitamin supplements.

The newspapers often report that food additives or artificial sweeteners cause cancer in animals, and some have been banned. It seems that there's always something new which can cause cancer - is this the case?

It's important that all additives, flavourings and colourings are investigated to find out if they are harmful. This research is carried out using animals and the substances are given in very high doses. There are two things to remember: the amount of additives used in these studies is much greater than we would normally take in during our entire lifetime, and also there are some differences in the way animals and human beings break down chemicals in the body.

New additives may only be used if there is no evidence that they cause cancer in human beings. If there is any chance, however small, then the substance is withdrawn from food manufacture.

There have been reports that all sorts of foods, from yoghurt to burnt or barbecued meat, can cause cancer. Is this true?

No. Once again there is no scientific evidence that either of these can cause cancer in human beings. Often small-scale laboratory studies are reported out of context and only serve to scare everyone. The best thing to do if you read any article like this is to check with your doctor who will be able to tell you if there is any truth in such a report or if it is just speculation.

It seems that a lot is written about a healthy diet but when it comes down to it nothing I do will make a difference to my cancer risk. Why should I bother to change?

We've already mentioned that eating more fruit and vegetables can reduce the risk of some cancers. However, although a link between diet and cancer generally has not been found, there are several other reasons why a well balanced diet is a good idea. We all need certain foods to keep our bodies healthy: protein to repair body tissues, carbohydrates and fats to give us energy, and fruit and vegetables to provide vitamins, minerals and roughage. The important point is to get the balance right. If we do this we will certainly reduce our risk of heart disease and we may also reduce the likelihood of developing cancer. Another plus is that we will usually keep our weight at a normal level and feel more attractive and comfortable.

What is a well balanced diet?

The current guidelines on healthy eating recommend that we

should cut down on the amount of fat we eat, particularly fatty meat and dairy products such as full cream milk. Alternatives like fish and chicken, skimmed milk and low fat spreads are easy to find in most supermarkets.

We should also cut down on sugar – eating a lot of sugar and sweet foods is one of the most common reasons for becoming overweight. Starchy foods, like bread, cereals and pasta, provide energy and are an important source of vitamins, minerals and fibre. The guidelines suggest we should eat more fruit and vegetables to increase our intake of vitamins, minerals and fibre, and we should reduce the amount of salt we use.

If you are worried about your weight or are unclear about what changes you need to make in order to eat a more healthy diet then your doctor or local health education unit will be able to advise you.

I've got a lot of information about healthy eating but I need some practical advice. Who should I go to?

Your doctor will be able to refer you to a dietitian, who will look at your individual lifestyle and advise you of any necessary changes.

I'm a vegetarian. Am I less likely to get cancer?

It is possible that your risk is reduced, as instead of eating meat you probably eat many of the foods recommended for a healthy diet, including plenty of fruit and vegetables. However, there is no guarantee because some forms of cancer are not associated with any dietary factors. For example, if you smoke or spend a lot of time sunbathing then being a vegetarian won't reduce your risk of lung or skin cancer.

For years people have said that getting out in the sun and fresh air is good for you. Now even this advice has changed. Does sunlight cause cancer?

Yes, prolonged exposure to sunlight or even a single episode of sunburn may cause skin cancer but this doesn't mean that you can't go out in the sun, it's just a question of common sense. There's no doubt that a sunny day makes us feel happier! We also need the vitamin D which is produced by a chemical reaction between our skin and the sun, although we can get some vitamin D in our diet. But these benefits have to be balanced against the risk of developing skin cancer – what we need is enough sun but not too much.

Are more people developing skin cancer now?

Yes. In the past skin cancer was most commonly seen in people who worked outside all their lives, for example sailors or farmers. Nowadays more people go abroad on holiday, especially to sunny resorts, and the incidence of skin cancers is rising. Most worrying is the increase in a particular type of skin cancer called **malignant melanoma** which, unlike other forms of skin cancer, can spread quickly to other parts of the body and can be fatal.

Isn't malignant melanoma the type of cancer that develops from moles?

Certainly most malignant melanomas develop from existing moles but not all do this. Perhaps not surprisingly people who have a great number of moles – or naevi – on their skin are at a higher risk of developing this type of skin cancer. If you have a mole that seems to suddenly change in some way such as by growing, changing shape or bleeding, or if you notice a new mole grow rapidly, then you should ask your doctor to check it and perhaps to remove it for your own peace of mind, even if it is thought unlikely to be cancerous.

What has damage to the ozone layer got to do with skin cancer?

There are two main types of ultraviolet radiation produced by the sun which reach the earth's surface: UVA and UVB. Both of these may be harmful to the skin but the most dangerous is UVB. Much UVB is removed by the protective ozone layer but if this layer is damaged these rays will reach the earth. The effects are not only destructive to the environment but may also increase the risk of skin cancer.

Who is most likely to get skin cancers from the sun?

Skin cancers are far more likely to occur in people who have fair skin and those who do not use sunblock creams or who allow themselves to burn in the sun. Children are particularly at risk of sunburn and should always be protected. Even people who tan easily should still take care not to overdo it in the sun when they have not been exposed to the sun's rays for some time and should at first use sun creams that have high protection factors in them. Black people should be aware that if they have not been out in strong sun for a while they, too, should use sun creams with higher protection factors at first.

What can I do to reduce my risk of developing skin cancer?

In Australia, fair-skinned people living in this very sunny climate have produced some sensible advice about limiting exposure to UV radiation. This is 'slip on a shirt, slop on some sun cream and slap on a hat'. Whenever possible stay in the shade but if you are in the sun, especially on holiday, increase the time you spend outside gradually day by day. Always take particular care during the hottest part of the day, wherever you are.

Does using a sunbed or sunlamp cause skin cancer?

It is difficult to say if using sunbeds or lamps cause skin cancer because most people who do also sunbathe. However, their use is not recommended – they may tan your skin but they can also cause it to age prematurely and, if you do not shield your eyes, you could develop problems such as cataracts.

If I'm worried about developing skin cancer and want to find out more about it, who should I contact?

Your doctor or local health education unit should be able to give you advice. Another helpful organisation is the **Cancer Research Campaign** which has produced a booklet called **Skin Cancer, The Sun and You: Your Questions Answered**. Their address is given in Appendix I.

As it appears that most of the enjoyable things in life can increase the risk of cancer, what about sex?

Ten or 20 years ago medical books stated that cancer of the cervix (neck of the womb) was never found in nuns but was common in prostitutes. This led to the belief that promiscuity and poor personal hygiene caused cancer. It is now known that there is a link between cervical cancer and a virus called the human papilloma virus, which may be passed between sexual partners. Having sexual intercourse doesn't cause cancer but the more partners you have the more you increase the chance of this virus being passed on to you. A simple way to prevent this is by using a condom, which can also protect you against other sexually transmitted diseases and AIDS (acquired immune deficiency syndrome).

Do viruses cause cancer?

Certain viruses have been shown by research to be linked with cancer. But these viruses don't actually cause cancer – instead they probably alter the body cells in some way so that there is a greater chance of cancer developing when another cancer-causing agent comes into contact with the cells.

Can you catch cancer from someone else?

No. There is no evidence that cancer is infectious or contagious like flu or measles.

People who have AIDS are more likely to develop cancer, aren't they?

The HIV virus which causes AIDS affects the immune system (the body's defence system) and therefore the body cannot fight infections or combat cells which go out of control and develop into cancers. People who have AIDS are at risk of getting certain rare cancers (such as Kaposi's sarcoma and lymphomas) but you cannot catch these cancers from them.

The HIV virus can only be passed on through body fluids such as blood and sperm. Guidance is widely available about ways in which you can reduce this risk, for example wearing a condom when you have sex.

Does the Pill cause cancer?

Many studies have been carried out to discover if taking an oral contraceptive pill does increase a woman's risk of developing cancer. The results have often been contradictory so we can only say that we don't know. Recent research has suggested that taking a pill which contains high levels of oestrogen for over eight years may slightly increase the risk of developing breast cancer in young women. However, today most women take low oestrogen pills or those containing no oestrogen at all. Doctors believe these are safe and that they may in fact provide protection against cancer of the ovary and endometrium (lining of the womb).

Does hormone replacement therapy (HRT) cause cancer?

This is another area where much research has been carried out and this is still continuing. The risk of developing cancer of the ovary or cancer of the cervix (neck of the womb) does not appear to be greater in women who take HRT. However, if a woman is taking an oestrogen-only preparation of HRT, then the risk of developing cancer of the uterus (womb) does rise. Combined hormone pills (which contain progesterone as well as oestrogen) are usually used to reduce this. The situation with regard to breast cancer is more complicated and there is a lot of discussion and disagreement between doctors. HRT probably does not cause breast cancer or, if it does increase the risk, then it does so only slightly. The benefits of HRT are beyond question, both in terms of relief from symptoms of the menopause and a reduction in heart disease or osteoporosis (thinning of the bones). Your doctor or an organisation like **Women's Health Concern** (address in Appendix I) will be able to offer advice.

How do I know if I'm at risk from cancer at work?

Several known carcinogens (cancer-causing substances) have been identified over the years, for example asbestos which causes a tumour called mesothelioma. Most of these substances or chemicals have been withdrawn from manufacturing processes. If this has not been possible and they are still in use, strict regulations have been laid down to control their usage and protect you, the employee. The **Health and Safety Executive** and the **Committee for Control of Substances Hazardous to Health** (COSHH) are the two main national bodies which can advise and help if you are concerned.

There must be lots of chemicals about which no one knows at the present time. What can I do if I'm worried about something I'm using?

One of the most important things to do is to wear all the recommended protective clothing offered to you at work and to follow all the procedures laid down by your employer. If you want to discuss this further talk to the occupational health department, works doctor, safety representative or your employer. If you're not happy with the answers you get you can contact your local office of the **Health and Safety Executive**, which will be listed in the phone book.

Everyone knows radiation causes cancer but it's all around us. How can we avoid exposure to it?

The short answer is 'we can't'. Natural radiation is present in the atmosphere and in the ground, and our doctors or dentists may ask for x-rays to check our health. Even putting all these sources together the amount of radiation we receive is very small and unlikely to do us any harm.

In parts of the UK, for example Cornwall and areas of Scotland, the level of radon gas, which is radioactive, is naturally higher. The **Department of the Environment** has produced a booklet called **The Householders' Guide to Radon** which provides guidance on how to reduce radon levels in your house and, therefore, your exposure to radiation.

What if I live near a power station, am I exposed to more radiation?

Only slightly: power stations (whatever fuel they use) release very small radiation doses into the atmosphere. We get only

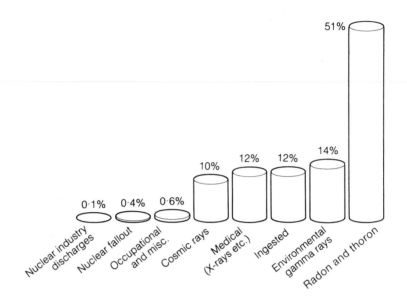

Figure 1: Sources of exposure to radiation.

a fraction of our very small annual exposure from power stations.

Workers in nuclear power stations and the rest of the nuclear industry are already well protected from overexposure, including monitoring procedures and regular medical checks. In addition, both the nuclear power industry and independent organisations are carrying out research to find out exactly what risks may, or may not, exist. If you are concerned you can contact your local office of the **Health and Safety Executive**, which will be listed in the phone book.

All this information about reducing risks applies to adults. Why do children get cancer?

The cause of the majority of childhood cancers is unknown. It is rare that a cancer is passed down through families: an example is retinoblastoma, an eye cancer, which accounts for 3% of all cancers in children (about 40 cases a year in the UK). Some cancers are more common in certain groups of children, such as acute leukaemia in those who have Down's syndrome. Research is continuing to discover if there is any common factor which can be identified in groups of children with specific cancers, or their families.

How many children develop cancer each year?

Childhood cancer is rare. About 1300 children in this country develop cancer each year. The number of children surviving for five and 10 years after their cancer has risen dramatically in the last 20 years. Overall about 50% of children are cured.

What can I do to prevent my child developing cancer?

There is no guarantee that your child will not develop cancer sometime in the future, maybe when they are 20, 30 or 40 years old. And you will not be able to influence their lifestyle - once they become adults it will be up to them to make choices about what they eat and how they behave. However, you may be able to dissuade them from taking up smoking, encourage them to eat a healthy diet and protect them from the sun, for example. You can also encourage them to be aware of their bodies and of any changes in their health so that they seek advice as soon as they notice anything which is not normal for them.

2

Symptoms, screening and investigations

Introduction

Generally the early diagnosis and treatment of cancer improves the prognosis (outcome). However, anxiety about a change in the body which may indicate cancer is present and fear of the disease often leads to a delay in someone contacting their doctor. The signs and symptoms of cancer are many and various so anything unusual should be reported as soon as possible to increase the chance of successful treatment.

Screening programmes for some cancers have been set up to enable early changes to be detected before any signs and symptoms develop. Pre-cancerous cells and very small tumours can be treated more effectively and the amount of treatment necessary is also reduced.

This chapter covers signs and symptoms, details of the screening programmes and self-examination and some of the more common tests which will be carried out to confirm or to exclude a diagnosis of cancer.

What are the signs or symptoms of cancer?

It is impossible to list the signs or symptoms which may indicate that cancer is present. Remember there are about 200 different types of cancer, affecting different organs or systems in the body. No one symptom means you may have cancer, it's a question of what is usual for you, and if something changes which concerns you, a visit to the doctor is necessary. You may worry needlessly if you do not have a check up. It is better that you find out what is wrong as soon as possible. The chances are it will not be cancer but, even if it is, the sooner it is treated the better the outcome.

The following are examples of the type of changes which you should take seriously if they persist for more than two weeks:

(i)   a change in bowel or bladder habits;

(ii)   a sore in the mouth or on the skin which does not heal;

(iii) any unusual bleeding or discharge from the vagina, back passage, bladder or nipple;

(iv) a thickening or lump in the breast, testicle or anywhere else in the body;

(v)   indigestion or difficulty in swallowing;

(vi) a noticeable change in a wart or mole (for example if it grows bigger or changes colour);

(vii) a nagging cough, hoarseness or loss of voice.

If a close friend or relative is worried about one of these signs, encourage them to go to the doctor.

I don't feel I can bother the doctor about something so trivial. He'll think I'm just being silly, won't he?

If something happens that worries you, it is not 'trivial'. Most doctors are very sympathetic and will listen to what you say, carry out a physical examination and either set your mind at rest immediately or refer you on for special tests if necessary.

I keep imagining I've got cancer every time I get an ache or pain. Have I got a cancer phobia?

One of the most common fears people have whenever they notice something unusual is that they have cancer. This doesn't mean you've got an irrational fear about cancer. Most of us are scared about changes in our health which we can't explain. Go and talk to your doctor. If she or he can't find anything wrong and you are still worried you may be able to talk with a counsellor, who may help you discover why you're so scared. There is usually a reason - perhaps someone close to you had cancer and died from it. The important point is that you talk about your fears and work out why you have them.

A woman friend of mine didn't have any of the listed symptoms, just a feeling of being uncomfortable and bloated in her tummy. The doctor said it was nothing but she died from cancer of the ovary. Why wasn't it found sooner?

Cancer of the ovary is, unfortunately, one of the 'silent' diseases. The ovary is a small organ in a large space so a cancer there can grow and spread without causing any symptoms. Ovarian cancer is the fifth most common cancer in the UK but it is still relatively rare – five times as many women develop breast cancer. Much research is currently being undertaken to try to detect cancer affecting organs deep inside the body at an earlier stage than is now possible. Both blood tests and ultrasound examinations (using sound waves) are being assessed as possible methods.

Diagnostic methods are not perfect and very often doctors have to consider many different possible causes for a problem, all of them more common than cancer.

If I'm just feeling unwell and tired, does it mean I could have cancer?

Possibly, but there are many other reasons too. All of us feel off-colour sometimes, and it usually means we've got flu or picked up a bug or been working too hard. However, if the symptoms continue for any length of time it's important to go to the doctor. If glands in your neck are enlarged too you might have an infection which needs treatment or you might need further tests to find out the cause of your fatigue.

Remember there are no specific signs or symptoms which mean you have cancer, and many of the symptoms of cancer can be associated with other illnesses. Whatever the situation it is important to contact your doctor and arrange for an examination for your own peace of mind and to make sure that any necessary treatment is received as soon as possible.

You read and hear about people who have knocked themselves or been injured when playing sports, then they're told they have cancer. Is the cancer caused by the knock?

No, there is no evidence that a knock or blow to any part of the body causes cancer. What usually happens is that the person feels that area of the body more carefully after an accident, and a lump which might have been present for a long time is suddenly noticed.

For a long time doctors told women to examine their breasts regularly, now they're saying the opposite. Should women still be looking for lumps?

Yes and no. It's very confusing when advice changes, or appears to change. 'Breast self-examination' has been replaced by 'breast awareness'. Awareness means becoming familiar with how your breasts feel and the changes that normally occur each month. For example, some women have tender, lumpy breasts just before their period.

By only feeling for lumps each month on the same day women could have been missing other changes which needed to be checked, such as changes in the skin colour or texture, alteration in the appearance of the nipple or discharge from it, and any unusual discomfort.

If you notice a lump or any change which is unusual for you, consult your family doctor or health clinic straight away.

There's been lots of recent publicity about testicular self-examination. Why - is testicular cancer becoming more common?

Yes, it is - in Britain, the USA, Denmark and New Zealand. There is no known reason for this increase. But treatment of testicular cancer is one of the success stories and over 90% of men who develop this type of cancer are cured.

This is why testicular self-examination is now recommended. Although only 1000 men, mainly in the 15–35 year old age range, develop the disease each year, the outlook is so good that doctors want to encourage anyone who finds a lump or notices hardening or swelling of a testicle to go to their family doctor straight away.

There seem to be so many 'don't knows' regarding cancer prevention and symptoms which might mean cancer is present - is it worth me having a regular medical examination?

Yes. You may find that your doctor or the practice nurse at your health centre already runs a 'Well Man' or 'Well Woman' clinic, or you can have an examination in your occupational health department at work. Organisations like BUPA in the independent health sector also provide these services. Women should definitely take advantage of the two free national screening programmes that exist, for cancer of the cervix and cancer of the breast.

What is the test for cancer of the cervix?

The test for cancer of the cervix (neck of the womb) is called a **smear** or **pap** test. The 'smear' refers to the layer of cells which is gently removed from the surface of the cervix using a small brush or wooden spatula. This is sent to the laboratory. We now know that these cells undergo a series of changes before they become cancerous. These changes are called cervical intra-epithelial neoplasia (CIN) or dysplasia (disordered cells). They are graded from 1 to 3, depending on how different they appear from the normal cells.

If abnormal cells are discovered at this **pre-cancerous** stage treatment is quick and easy, and may be given as an out-patient. A laser may be used to kill the cells or part of the cervix may be removed during an operation.

How do I get a smear test?

If you are between 20 and 64 years old you should receive an invitation from your family doctor to go for a test. If you have not been invited, or did not attend when you were first asked, make an appointment to see your doctor or the practice nurse, who may often run a special clinic. You should attend even if you are a virgin, are not having sexual intercourse or have had your menopause (change of life).

Once you have been for one test you will automatically be recalled at least every five years and often more frequently, for example at three year intervals. It will depend on the routine in your area.

If I'm asked to go back for another test straight away does it mean I've got cancer?

No. Sometimes there may not be enough cells in the original sample and the laboratory will ask for another smear to be taken. Even if you're told the test is positive it doesn't mean cancer is present. Remember, the doctors are looking for pre-cancerous changes so they can offer you treatment and prevent cancer from developing.

Is cancer of the cervix preventable?

In one sense, yes. We don't know exactly what causes the cells to change but if every woman had regular cervical smears the abnormal cells could probably be treated before cancer develops.

The Breast Screening Programme is quite new. Why has it been set up?

The Breast Screening Programme has been established to try to reduce the number of women who die each year from breast cancer. In the United Kingdom and many other developed countries breast cancer is the most common type of malignancy. Research has shown that treatment is much more successful if a cancer is discovered when it is small or when it is **pre-clinical**, that is before a lump in the breast can be felt. A special x-ray of the breast called a **mammogram** can detect very small lumps or areas of abnormal cells.

Why are only women over 50 eligible for breast screening?

First of all because breast cancer is much more common in older women. Secondly, because the breast tissue is more dense in younger women, which means it is difficult to tell which is a normal area of thickening and which is an abnormal area. If younger women were screened routinely they would probably end up having many unnecessary investigations, which would cause a great deal of anxiety.

If I'm the right age for screening, will I be called to have a mammogram?

Yes. You should receive an invitation from your family doctor or direct from the screening clinic. You should also be sent an information leaflet which will answer some of the questions you may have about the screening procedure. If you are over 65 you may make an appointment at the screening clinic yourself, as at the present time you will not be automatically invited. If you are younger and there is a history of breast cancer in your family, you may be called for an ultrasound test.

How often are the mammograms repeated?

Every three years. However, if you are concerned about a change in your breasts between screening appointments you should contact your doctor.

How do I find out if my x-ray is normal?

The results of your mammogram will be sent to you and your doctor.

If I'm called back for a repeat mammogram, does it mean I've got cancer?

Not necessarily. Most abnormalities seen on a mammogram are benign lumps, such as cysts (fluid-filled lumps). Sometimes a repeat x-ray is needed because there was a technical problem and the picture is not clear. It is important that you attend your second appointment so this can be checked. If further investigations or treatment are necessary these can then be carried out as soon as possible.

Isn't it true that even if I change my personal habits and have all these checks I might still get cancer if I have a cancer personality?

The theory that there is a cancer-prone personality goes back many centuries but even now the answer is not clear. Some researchers and psychologists believe that there is a connection between personality and cancer development, and also with heart disease. Others believe equally strongly that there is no link whatsoever and that cancer is a purely physical disorder. The answer is probably somewhere in between and more research is needed before it is possible to say that a particular type of person or personality may be more likely to get cancer (and why!) and to know what we can do to prevent it.

Does stress cause cancer?

There is no evidence that stress can increase the risk of developing cancer.

Why do many people appear to develop cancer after stressful events, such as a bereavement or a divorce?

We know that cancer usually takes many years to develop, so it appears unlikely it could be related to an event in the immediate past. However, researchers are continuing to study people with cancer to discover if there could be a connection. One explanation may be that when people are very stressed and anxious, for whatever reason, they are less concerned with their physical health. It is then only after a crisis has passed that they notice a sign or symptom which leads them to consult a doctor. There is still some controversy about whether stress can speed up changes in cells and research is continuing into this theory.

If my doctor suspects I might have cancer what happens next?

Your doctor will ask you several questions to put together your medical history and will also perform a physical examination. During this time the doctor will concentrate on the sign or symptom about which you are complaining. Various tests or investigations may be asked for by your doctor so that any other causes can be eliminated. Examples of symptoms with causes other than cancer are:

(i)   if you are short of breath, you may have a chest infection;
(ii) if you have difficulty passing urine, you may have an infection in your bladder;
(iii) if you are bleeding from your rectum (back passage) you may have haemorrhoids (piles); or

(iv) if you are feeling tired and run down you may be anaemic,
     and need some extra iron.

When the doctor has examined you and received the results of
any tests, the conclusion may be that a diagnosis of cancer is the
possible cause for your symptoms. If this is so you will be
referred to the hospital and the care of a specialist.

What kind of specialist will I go to?

This will depend on what kind of cancer your doctor suspects
you may have. If you are having problems with your bowel it will
probably be a surgeon; if there is an abnormality with your
blood, you will be referred to a haematologist, who specialises in
treatment of blood disorders.

Does every hospital have a cancer specialist?

No. Many hospitals have a surgeon or physician who has a
special interest in a particular type of cancer and every health
authority has a regional radiotherapy (radiation treatment) or
oncology (tumour) centre, often in the major town or city. Your
specialist will usually refer you to one of these units after
diagnosis or if a specific treatment is indicated for you. There
are also specialist children's cancer treatment centres throughout the country, and other units which offer expert care during
bone marrow transplant, for example. In some areas, such as
London, there may be several radiotherapy and oncology units.

How will the doctor make a diagnosis of cancer?

In order to be certain that you have cancer and, especially,
exactly what type of cancer you might have, a **biopsy** (sample of
tissue) must be obtained and sent to the laboratory for
examination under the microscope.

Will I always have to go into hospital for an operation?

No. There are several ways of obtaining this tissue sample, some
of these can be performed in an out-patient clinic and some
require you to be admitted to hospital. The following list
explains the most common procedures.

(i)   The suspicious lump or abnormal area may be completely removed - for example, a lymph gland or an ulcer on the skin.

(ii)   A sample of cells may be taken from a deeper lump using a special biopsy needle - for example, from a breast lump.

(iii)   A scope (a flexible or stiff tube) may be passed into part of your body and a small piece of tissue removed using long forceps - for example, a gastroscope may be passed into your stomach or a cystoscope into your bladder.

(iv)   Cells may be aspirated (drawn off) using a needle and syringe - this is a common way of obtaining cells from a breast lump.

(v)   Cells may be drawn from your bone marrow, usually from your hip bone, if it is suspected you may have leukaemia.

(vi)   You may be asked to provide a specimen of urine or sputum (phlegm) and this can be examined to discover if any cancer cells are present.

(vii)   A smear of cells may be removed from your cervix using a small brush or wooden spatula.

Are these procedures painful?

Some methods of obtaining cells are not painful and some are just uncomfortable for a brief moment. If the procedure is likely to cause any pain or distress you will be offered an anaesthetic or sedation, that is an injection or tablet to make you sleepy.

The type of anaesthetic may vary. You may only need a **local** anaesthetic, when sensation is removed from a specific area of your body, or you may have a **general** anaesthetic, where you are asleep throughout the whole procedure. Whatever is planned for you will be explained by the doctors and nurses.

If cancer is confirmed, what other investigations will I have?

Any investigations or tests will depend on what type of cancer you have. The next six questions discuss some of the most common tests and you may have some or all of these. But there may be some extra less common tests which are not explained here. The important thing is that you should understand what a test involves and why it is being done. If you don't understand, or you don't remember what you were told the first time, ask again.

Why might I have blood tests?

Blood samples are taken to assess your general health and how certain organs in your body are functioning, for example your liver or kidneys. Sometimes they may be able to provide information about your current illness, for example leukaemia, which affects the blood cells. If the doctor thinks you might need a blood transfusion before or during treatment a blood sample will be taken to discover your blood group. Blood will usually be taken from a vein in your arm using a needle and syringe or a special vacuum tube.

What shows up on an x-ray?

An x-ray is a picture of organs inside your body taken by a special machine. On a chest x-ray the doctors can see if your heart and lungs are healthy, look at the lymph nodes in your chest and check that there are no tumours in your lungs. You may be asked to have more extensive x-rays, for example of your bones, or more complicated investigations to outline your internal organs. Any special procedures will be explained to you. Do ask questions if there is anything you don't understand.

I've got to have an ultrasound scan. Isn't that what pregnant women have?

Yes. An ultrasound scan uses sound waves to obtain pictures of a baby in the womb and can also be used to see internal organs such as your liver. The ultrasound waves are sent to and from your body by moving a special sensor (similar to a microphone) over the surface of your skin in the area to be examined. A gel will be spread on to your skin to help conduct the waves. Ultrasound bounces back from various structures in the body and a picture is formed on a television screen. The procedure is painless.

What are isotope scans?

An isotope is a radioactive substance, and certain isotopes are attracted to different organs in the body. When a very small quantity of an isotope is injected into a vein, usually in your arm or hand, it travels around your body and is taken up by the 'target' organ. Then, when you are asked to lie or stand in front of a special camera detailed and clear pictures of parts of your body can be obtained. Isotope scans may be used to examine your bones, brain, thyroid and many other organs. The scan is painless. The amount of radioactivity you receive is not harmful and your body quickly excretes it.

What's the difference between a CT scan and an x-ray?

The CT scanner is a complicated x-ray machine that uses a computer to produce pictures which resemble 'slices' through different parts of your body. You will be asked not to eat or drink for four hours before the scan. A CT scan is not harmful or painful but you will have to lie still for up to an hour. The table on which you lie is hard so this may be uncomfortable. The table moves through the x-ray part of the machine as you are being scanned and comes out the other side so you may feel closed in temporarily. You may also have an injection of 'contrast' (dye) given into a vein in your arm or hand. You should feel no effects from this. The purpose of the contrast is to provide clearer images of certain organs.

What is an MR scan?

An MR scan machine uses a magnetic field to build up extremely detailed pictures of the body. The full name for this investigation is **magnetic resonance imaging**. Computers and radio waves are also used but no radioactive substances. There is usually no special preparation. Not everyone can have this type of scan, for example it is not suitable for people who have metal in their body such as a heart pacemaker. You also cannot take certain things into the scanning room, for example keys and watches. Before you come for the scan you may be asked to wear clothes which do not have metal fastenings (for example zips) or you might be asked to change into a gown when you arrive. The scan is not harmful or painful but you will have to lie still for about an hour which may be uncomfortable. The table on which you lie moves into the scanning machine and so you may feel closed in temporarily. You may have an injection of 'contrast' (dye) given into a vein in your arm or hand in order to provide clearer pictures of certain organs. You should feel no effects from this.

Why do different people have different tests even if they have the same diagnosis?

Each person is different and the doctors will ask for the specific investigations which provide most information about you. Don't be alarmed if you have some tests and not others, or if you have an investigation which no-one else is having. Certain scans, for example, may not be a helpful aid to diagnosis in your particular case.

Are the tests just done once or will I have to have them again?

All the tests you have may be repeated during your treatment or even before any decisions are made. This may be because of technical problems or because a result is borderline between normal and abnormal. There are all sorts of reasons, such as comparing results before and after treatment. Having a test repeated does not mean that your condition is more serious than expected.

How long do all these tests take?

The time you may be at the hospital for tests varies. A chest x-ray or blood test may be over in minutes and a scan may take an hour. Occasionally the preparation for an investigation may take longer than the procedure itself, or you may have to attend more than once during a day. An example of this is an isotope scan: you are given an injection but may have to wait a couple of hours before you have the scan because it takes time for the isotope to circulate round your body.

Always ask for details of tests, including the time they take or the time you have to wait. You may wish to take a friend with you, or a book to read.

How long does it take to get the results of all these tests?

It varies. Some test results can be available almost immediately, such as a simple blood test or a routine chest x-ray. But very often the results take days or a couple of weeks to reach your doctor. Take a scan as an example – the person performing the scan can identify the parts of your body but the pictures produced must be carefully interpreted by a specialist doctor who will write a report and send it to your doctor. This is bound to take a few days.

The waiting is the worst. Is there anything I can do?

Many people find this time the most difficult. It's a time of uncertainty and fear and all the people caring for you know this. You may find it helps to talk to your doctor or to the nurses in a ward or clinic or to your family doctor. It's also going to be an anxious time for your family. It may help to discuss your fears and concerns with those close to you.

There are also organisations who can provide a listening ear, positive support and additional information. It may help to talk to people who don't know you well, such as those in a support group or someone on the end of a telephone. Organisations which offer such help are listed in Appendix I.

What happens next?

When your doctor has all the results of your tests, she or he will be able to advise you about what treatments are available, what alternatives exist and what is your best course of action. It is important that you understand what is said, what is being offered and that you ask all the questions you want. Take a friend or relative with you when you go to see your doctor, make notes and if you want time to think about what has been said, don't be afraid to ask for it. It's not uncommon to have difficulty taking in all the information immediately, so don't feel stupid if you ask about things more than once.

What treatment will I have?

There are several ways of treating cancer and your treatment will be planned individually for you. The treatment recommended will depend on many factors: the type of cancer, the degree of spread, your age and general health, to name a few. Do not be concerned if you speak to people who are having similar, but different, treatments. Always ask your doctor or anyone caring for you about your personal treatment as she or he will be able to explain exactly what is planned and why. If it takes a little time to make a decision or for treatment to be organised, don't worry. Cancer doesn't usually get worse in a few weeks.

3
Treatment and care

Introduction

When all the results of your tests and investigations have been received, your doctor will be able to advise you about what sort of treatment you should have. There are five main types of treatment for cancer – surgery, radiotherapy, chemotherapy, hormone therapy and biological therapy. Each of these may be used alone although it is more common to have a combination of two or more types of treatment. The choice of which treatment or which combination is recommended for you will depend on whether the cancer is confined to one organ or area of the body, or if it has spread. The aim of treatment may be to cure the person with cancer or to control the disease.

Your doctor should offer you an opportunity to discuss your planned treatment and ask questions about it before a decision is made. It is important that you understand what the treatment involves before you agree to it. Your consent is needed before starting any treatment and similarly you may refuse treatment if you so wish.

Can cancer be cured?

Yes, at least one in three people who develop cancer will be cured, although the likelihood of cure varies from cancer to cancer. For example, skin cancers are easy to see and very rarely spread to other parts of the body (with the exception of melanoma). They can be treated simply by removing them so the cure rate is over 95%. Another good example is testicular cancer which responds very well to drug treatment: the cure rate is over 90%. An increasing number of children's cancers are curable.

Unfortunately, some of the most common cancers cannot always be cured but of these many can be controlled by treatment. It is possible for people to live for several years with their disease under control without undue impact on their daily activities.

What do doctors mean when they talk about survival rates?

Doctors are very cautious people. They often cannot say whether or not they have been able to remove all the cancer and cure the patient, because many cancers spread to other parts of the body and lie there undetected for several years. So doctors use phrases like three year, five year and 10 year survival rates, based on the percentage of people who are likely to be alive that long after their diagnosis and treatment. Some of these people may be known to still have cancer in their bodies but they are alive and living with their cancer. Others may have no detectable cancer at that time but doctors still hesitate to use the word 'cure' because certain cancers have been known to reappear 15 or 20 years later.

I've got bladder cancer and I've been told there's a 60% chance of surviving five years. What does this mean to me?

You can only use the figure given to you by your doctor as a rough guide. No-one can know whether you will be one of the people who make up the 60% when the statistics are reviewed in five years time.

National statistics are gathered on all the people who are treated for bladder cancer. When they are analysed after five years, 60% of those people are still alive while 40% have died because of their cancer or from other causes. The problem with statistics is they don't take account of your individual case and this means that even if you know you have a 60% chance of survival there will always be some uncertainty.

What kind of things affect the chances of being cured of, or of surviving cancer?

First of all, the type of cancer you have – remember there are over 200 different kinds. Secondly, whether the cancer has been picked up at an early stage before it has had an opportunity to spread; and lastly, what effective treatment is available for your particular cancer.

Surgery

Most cancers are treated by an operation, aren't they?

Whenever possible doctors try to remove the whole tumour and this may mean the affected organ is taken out. Surgery is commonly used for cancer of the skin, stomach, bowel, uterus (womb), breast and testicle. It may also be used to remove cancers in the face and neck region, including the thyroid gland and larynx, and cancers of the ovary and prostate.

It is important that all the cancer is removed so a large operation is often needed, which may cause disfigurement or a change in body function. The lymph glands in the area around the tumour are usually the first place to which a cancer spreads. These are frequently removed during the same operation.

Does everyone have an operation?

Most people with cancer have an operation at some time during their treatment but the purpose of the operation may be different in individual situations. For example, an operation may be performed simply to obtain a biopsy (tissue sample), or it might be the primary treatment to remove the cancer, or surgery may be used to relieve symptoms at a later stage such as those caused by a blockage due to a secondary cancer.

When someone is told that a tumour is inoperable, what does it mean?

Inoperable means that the cancer cannot be surgically removed. This may be because the cancer has spread to adjoining organs, or because it is situated in a organ like the brain, and to remove it might cause damage to normal tissue. It may be possible to remove part of a tumour to enable easier and more effective treatment by another form of therapy, such as radiotherapy. If the cancer is causing troublesome symptoms, a 'bypass' operation may be performed to relieve these. For example, jaundice and itching associated with cancer of the pancreas may be relieved by a bypass which takes pressure off the gallbladder. This allows bile, which causes these symptoms, to drain freely again into the bowel.

The fact that a cancer is inoperable does not mean that it is untreatable. But it may mean that a cancer cannot be cured, only controlled by other therapies.

I've heard that when you have an operation for cancer it increases the risk of the cancer spreading. Is this true?

There is no evidence that the risk of cancer cells spreading is increased by surgery to remove the original tumour.

Is cutting a cancer out the only way to cure it?

No. For certain cancers the primary and most effective treatment is an operation to remove it. For others either an operation or radiotherapy (radiation treatment) may be equally good treatments, for example for cancers of the skin or larynx (voice box). And in some malignancies, like lymphomas and leukaemias, the first and best treatment may be radiotherapy or chemotherapy (drug treatment). Using these alone or in combination can also produce cures.

When my father had treatment for cancer years ago it was so straightforward. He had an operation and it was all over very quickly. Now treatment seems to take longer and it's much more complicated. Why?

Basically the doctors know a great deal more about cancer and how to treat it than they used to, and they have a wider range of treatments they can use. Sometimes an operation is still the only treatment necessary but with many cancers the cure and survival rates can be increased greatly by giving post-operative radiotherapy and/or chemotherapy. Radiotherapy may be the primary (first-line) treatment, followed by anti-cancer drugs or vice versa. These treatments must be given over a period of weeks or months in order to be most effective and to reduce side effects.

Is there a special name for this type of therapy?

Yes. Doctors call this way of giving treatment **adjuvant** therapy.

How do the doctors decide if adjuvant therapy is necessary?

For every type of cancer there is a sophisticated system of assessing the extent of the disease: that is whether it is confined to one organ or part of the body, if it has spread to the nearby lymph glands or if there are secondaries (metastases) in distant sites. This is called **staging**. Even if there is no evidence of widespread cancer, the doctors know that some types of cancer are more likely than others to spread. They use adjuvant therapy as an insurance policy, to reduce the chance of this happening in the future. For example, after an operation radiotherapy may be given to the nearby lymph glands which are often the first place to which cancer cells spread. Alternatively drugs may be administered after radiotherapy, and these travel around the whole body seeking out cancer cells in other places.

When a person has a malignant disease which affects tissue found throughout the body, such as Hodgkin's disease (which affects the lymph glands) or leukaemia (which affects the bone marrow and blood cells), it is called a **systemic** disease. Chemotherapy, a systemic treatment, is the first-line, most effective way of treatment.

What does stage I disease mean?

Stage I means that a cancer or malignancy has been diagnosed early when it is limited to one part of the body. When a cancer is widespread it is referred to as stage IV. There are precise, internationally agreed criteria which doctors use to determine the stage of the disease and this usually guides what the treatment will be.

How do doctors know what stage a disease is at?

By studying the results of all the investigations which have been carried out. If someone's treatment was started before the tests were done it is possible that in some cases they would not receive the most effective treatment.

How do I know if I need an operation?

You have to trust the opinion of your doctors. Ask them what the operation will involve, what the alternative treatments are and what effect the surgery will have on you. In many instances there may be one operation which the majority of surgeons agree is the most effective for your condition. However, sometimes the experts disagree which is why you should have an opportunity to discuss the pros and cons. If you are still unhappy with what is proposed you can always ask for a second opinion from another doctor. Some people find this reassuring if the recommended treatment is the same, but it may be confusing if it is different.

A lot depends on your relationship with your own surgeon and how willing she or he is to discuss the operation with you, and allow you time to decide.

How do I know that what I agree to have done is what will actually happen?

Before your operation your surgeon should explain exactly what she or he proposes to do and why. You will then be asked to sign a consent form which shows that you agree to the operation. In law, the surgeon can only carry out the procedure to which you have consented, unless an emergency arises during the operation and an immediate change of plan is required. If such a situation should arise, the surgeon must explain to you what happened and what needed to be done. If you are not satisfied with this explanation you are entitled to make a formal complaint.

I had prepared myself for a big operation but when I came back from the operating theatre, the surgeon said it wasn't possible to remove my cancer. Why couldn't he have told me before?

It is very disappointing when you have prepared yourself physically and emotionally for something which doesn't happen. However, it is not uncommon. Despite all the careful investigations carried out beforehand, the surgeon may often not know the exact situation until the operation starts. If the cancer is more widespread than it appeared it may not be possible to remove it because it is affecting other organs. An alternative operation may be necessary or a completely different type of treatment may be needed instead.

What will happen before my operation for cancer?

Exactly what will happen depends on where your cancer is and what operation you are going to have. It is only possible to give general information, as procedures may also differ from hospital to hospital.

You will usually be admitted a few days before your operation so that you can become familiar with your surroundings. Any necessary tests can be carried out, or repeated. Special preparation may be needed before some surgery, for example to ensure the bowel is empty prior to an operation which reduces the risk of an infection afterwards. This preparation may take one or two days to complete. You will meet the doctors, nurses and others caring for you, such as specialist nurses, dietitians or physiotherapists. You will have the opportunity to ask them any questions you may have about your personal treatment.

The days before an operation are a time of anxiety for most people. It is quite normal for you to be worried about what is about to happen and what the outcome will be. It can help to talk about your concerns with the staff caring for you – they may be able to assist in a variety of ways and sometimes just sharing your feelings helps. Always remember that there are other people in the hospital who may be able to support you in different ways, for example the chaplain (representatives of many faiths or religions work in or visit hospitals) or the social worker if you are worried about your job or your finances.

What will happen after my operation?

This is a difficult question to answer except in general terms.

When surgery is used as the primary (first-line) treatment for cancer, a large operation may be necessary. After the operation you will need extra medical and nursing care and will probably be looked after in a small special ward or unit. The nurses will take your pulse and blood pressure frequently to monitor your condition. You may have a mask over your mouth and nose to give you oxygen to help you to recover from the anaesthetic.

Everyone experiences pain in different ways. The amount of pain or discomfort also varies depending on the operation you have had. Hopefully you will not feel too sore or uncomfortable but if you do you should tell your nurse straight away so you can be given some analgesia (painkillers). Also tell the nurse if you are feeling sick, so that you can be given an anti-emetic (anti-sickness) drug.

When you wake up you may have various tubes in place. All of these have a particular function. Some patients will have an intravenous infusion (an IV 'drip'). A cannula (fine tube) is placed into a vein in your arm, or occasionally into a vein in your neck. Fluids, and any drugs which you need, can be administered through this while you are recovering from your operation. Once you can take fluids by mouth again the infusion will be discontinued. The time before you are able to drink and eat normally will vary from a day to over a week depending on your operation.

Some people will have a catheter (tube) in the bladder to drain urine away. This will not be left in place any longer than necessary.

A tube may have been passed into your stomach to remove natural secretions which collect there and which may make you feel sick. This is passed down your nose and will not affect your ability to speak. The secretions may drain into a bag or the nurses may draw them off from time to time using a syringe.

It is normal for blood and fluid to be produced when any tissue has been cut. A wound drain (another tube) will usually be in place to remove this fluid from your operation site. This will be removed after a few days.

These are some of the common things to expect. You may

experience all or some of them, or there may be other procedures which are special to you. If you do not understand what is happening and why, ask the staff caring for you.

When the doctors are satisfied with your progress you will return to your own ward.

I have breast cancer and my surgeon says I don't need to have my breast removed, but surely mastectomy is always safer, isn't it?

Not necessarily: research has shown that a smaller operation such as lumpectomy (removal of the lump only) followed by radiotherapy can be just as effective as a mastectomy for many women. Mastectomy may be the best treatment for some breast cancers and some women prefer it because they want to be sure all the cancer has been physically removed.

Nowadays, most surgeons will try to preserve the breast if at all possible, and only remove the lump or part of the breast.

Can I have a new breast created?

Yes. There are a number of techniques used for breast reconstruction, using muscle from other parts of the body such as the shoulder or using a breast implant. More information can be found in a booklet called **Breast Reconstruction**. Details of this booklet can be found in Appendix II.

After all the recent publicity, are breast implants safe?

Probably. The Department of Health and many experts in the use of implants have considered the available evidence. They have stated publicly that there is no reason to stop using implants for reconstructive surgery. As with any 'foreign body' implanted into the human body there is a possibility of rejection or infection. If you are considering having an implant at the time of your breast surgery, or at a later date, discuss the procedure and its advantages and disadvantages with your surgeon. If you have had a breast implant and are at all worried, speak to your surgeon.

If I have a mastectomy, will I look different afterwards?

There is no reason why your appearance, when dressed, should be any different from before your operation. You will be fitted with a prosthesis, an artificial breast form, which will be similar in size, shape and weight to your own breast. This cannot be fitted until after your wound has healed and so you will be given a light temporary prosthesis at first, before you leave hospital. An appointment will be made for a permanent prosthesis to be fitted about six weeks after your operation. If a course of radiotherapy is planned for you, this fitting may be delayed because your skin may become sensitive or sore during the treatment.

My dentist found a small ulcer in my mouth which the specialist says is a cancer. The operation that is planned is much bigger than I thought would be necessary to remove such a small ulcer. Why?

The surgeon will want to make sure that all the cancer has been removed. She or he will want to cut out an area of normal tissue around the ulcer and also to remove nearby lymph glands to which the cancer may have spread. The surgeon may also need to remove some of the skin over or around the tumour and to replace it with a skin graft from another part of your body. All this does mean an extensive operation but if the cancer is not removed it will continue to grow. If it is not completely removed there is a strong possibility that it will recur (return) in the same area and it may not be possible to treat it so effectively. It is important that you talk about the operation and what it entails with the doctors, nurses and others who will be caring for you. They will be able to explain what will happen and why it is necessary for you.

If I have an operation on my mouth or throat, will I look different?

Not necessarily: sometimes all the surgery can be carried out from inside the mouth and then there are no external scars, or scarring is minimal. However, your appearance may be altered quite markedly and there may be a lot of scarring.

Even if this has been explained to you before your operation, you may still be distressed when you first look at your face. Scarring and puffiness will lessen over time and cosmetic camouflage techniques can be used to make scars less noticeable. If any facial bones need to be removed during the operation a special prosthesis, a lightweight false bone, will be made individually for you. There is an organisation for people who have had surgery to the face called **Let's Face It** – the address is given in Appendix I.

I have cancer of the larynx and am going to have my voice-box removed. Will I be able to talk after the operation?

Not immediately. Instead you will have to use a pen and paper to communicate with the doctors, nurses, your family and friends. But you should be able to talk again in as little as six weeks, depending on which technique of voice restoration is suitable for you.

Before your operation you will meet a speech and language therapist who will explain the various ways of regaining your voice. She or he will work closely with you after your laryngectomy (removal of the voice-box) to help you speak again.

The operation itself and the different methods of voice restoration (for example special valves and developing an oesophageal voice) are explained in a booklet **Laryngectomy** and you can find out more from the **National Association of Laryngectomee Clubs**. Details of how to obtain the booklet and how to contact this organisation are given in Appendix II and Appendix I.

What's the difference between a stoma and a colostomy?

A stoma is an artificial opening onto the skin. There are different types of stomas that are named after the parts of the body which are used to form them. For example a **tracheostomy** is formed from the trachea (windpipe) and an **ileostomy** is formed from the ileum (small bowel). A **colostomy** is a stoma formed from the colon (large bowel).

Why do some people with bowel cancer have a colostomy while others don't?

Often when a person develops bowel cancer the surgeon can resect (cut out) the tumour and stitch the two ends of normal bowel back together. When the cancer is near the rectum (back passage) this may not be possible, even using the most up-to-date techniques. If there is not enough remaining bowel to join together after a resection then a colostomy is formed. This provides an alternative, artificial opening to enable the stools (faeces) to leave the body. You will need to wear a special unobtrusive bag (appliance) to collect your stools.

Are there different kinds of colostomy?

Yes, sometimes a colostomy is permanent and at others it is temporary. A temporary colostomy may be formed to relieve a blockage in the bowel until normal function can be resumed. The blockage may be caused by a cancer in another organ close to the bowel, for example the ovary. Treatment for this cancer may relieve the blockage which means the colostomy can be 'closed' and bowel function becomes normal again.

If you are told that you may have a colostomy formed, ask for more details from your surgeon. Many hospitals have a specialist stoma care nurse who will be able to provide more information, practical help and support. The **British Colostomy Association** can also help. Their address is in Appendix I.

Is an operation for cancer always a big operation which causes disfigurement or a change in how the body works?

No. For example, the majority of bladder cancers which affect only the lining of the bladder can be completely removed through a cystoscope (a tube passed into the bladder) without affecting the way it works. Regular check ups are carried out and, even if the cancer returns, it may be possible to remove it once again in the same way.

Will an operation for cancer mean I can't have children?

It may do. Certainly if a woman has her ovaries or uterus

(womb) removed as treatment for cancer of the ovary, uterus or cervix she will not be able to have children.

If a man has an orchidectomy (removal of one testicle) it does not mean he will be infertile or impotent and unable to father children. The remaining testicle will continue to produce sperm and intercourse is still possible.

Always ask if the operation planned for you affects your reproductive organs, or organs close by.

If an adult or child has a bone tumour does it always mean they have to have an amputation?

Not always. A bone tumour is a good example of a situation where combination (adjuvant) therapy can reduce the size or type of operation required. Obviously the tumour must be removed but if it can be reduced in size by chemotherapy (drug treatment) then a smaller piece of bone can be removed and replaced by a metal prosthesis (false part). This avoids the need for an amputation.

Radiotherapy

Can radiotherapy be used instead of an operation?

Yes. A course of radiotherapy may be given in place of an operation, particularly if a cancer is situated deep inside the body or in an organ such as the brain. The outcome may be just as good and the function of the organ may not be affected. However, as with all treatment for cancer, the decision about which treatment is better and why is made after an assessment of each individual case.

What is radiotherapy?

Radiotherapy is the use of high energy rays to kill cancer cells in the part of the body being treated. X-rays may be used, or treatment may be given by using gamma rays produced by a radioactive source. Cancer cells are more sensitive to radio-therapy than normal cells and will be killed at a greater rate.

Any normal cells that are affected recover or repair themselves quite quickly.

But radiation can cause cancer, how can it be used to treat it?

When radiation is used in therapy it is very carefully controlled. The beam of rays is directed exactly to the area needing treatment. The dose of radiation is small and is given over a period of weeks.

Is radiotherapy painful?

No. The treatment is entirely painless.

How is radiotherapy given?

Radiotherapy is given in one of two ways. **External** radiotherapy uses machines that produce x-rays or gamma rays. A beam of rays is directed at the cancer. Occasionally an applicator fitted onto the end of the machine will touch you gently but usually it is some distance away. This is the most common method of delivering radiotherapy.

Internal radiotherapy involves placing a radioactive 'source' inside the body. This may take the form of tubes placed in a body cavity (such as the vagina) or the sources may be inside fine needles which are inserted into the tumour area. You will be given an anaesthetic to prevent discomfort when the sources are inserted and probably when they are removed. During the time they are in place you will not feel any sensations from the radiation itself.

Why are different methods of radiotherapy used?

The method of giving radiotherapy depends on the type of cancer and where it is situated. External radiotherapy is the method most commonly used. Internal radiotherapy has the advantage that the treatment can be concentrated in the area where it is most needed. Sometimes an internal treatment is all that is necessary but often it is used with external therapy to give a top-up or boost to a specific part of the treatment area. Gynaecological tumours, for example cancer of the cervix, may be treated in this way.

A friend of mine with thyroid cancer had a radioactive drink. Is this is a type of radiotherapy?

Yes. The drink was radioactive iodine which is used to treat thyroid diseases and some forms of thyroid cancer. Iodine is necessary for the normal working of the thyroid gland and is attracted specifically to it. When thyroid cells are overactive, or become cancerous, a radioactive form of iodine can be given as treatment. Like ordinary iodine, the radioactive iodine is taken up by the thyroid cells. The radioactivity painlessly destroys them.

This is an uncommon way to give radiotherapy, as there are very few cancers which can be treated in this way.

Am I radioactive during a course of radiotherapy?

No, not if you are having external radiotherapy. The machine is switched on for the treatment time and switched off afterwards. There is no radiation left in you or in the air around you when the machine has been switched off at the end of your treatment.

If you have internal therapy you will be temporarily radio-active while the 'source' is inside your body. Once this has been removed at the end of your treatment you are no longer carrying any radiation.

If you have radioiodine therapy, your body will take a few days to get rid of the radioactivity. There will be restrictions on what you can do during this period and on the time others may spend with you.

Do I need to be admitted to hospital for radiotherapy?

Not usually. Most people have radiotherapy as an out-patient. Some particular treatments do require admission. If you have internal radiotherapy you may have to stay in hospital, probably in a side room, for the duration of your treatment. Ask the staff caring for you exactly what your treatment plan involves.

How long does radiotherapy last? Will I just have one treatment?

Radiotherapy is usually given as a course of treatment over 4–6

weeks, but this may vary depending on what your radio-
therapist (the doctor who specialises in radiation treatment)
recommends for you. You will usually be asked to attend for
treatment each day from Monday to Friday. Sometimes treatments are only given once or twice a week and occasionally they
are given more than once a day. Ask what is planned for you. The
treatment only lasts for a few minutes but before each treatment you, and the machine, have to be carefully placed in the
right position by the radiographers. This often takes longer than
the treatment itself.

**Now I've been told I have to have radiotherapy I want to get
on with it, but there seems to be so much planning to do.
Why?**

It is essential that the radiotherapy beam is accurately directed
at the area to be treated. The area may be the cancer itself, or a
region of the body to which cancer cells may have spread, for
example lymph glands. During treatment planning a special
machine called a **simulator** is used. This creates a mock-up of
treatment and helps to make sure that all the area which needs
to be treated is in the treatment 'field' and also that no normal
tissue is being treated unnecessarily.

The planning phase may vary in length and may require more
than one visit to the simulator. This is an important part of your
radiotherapy so try to be patient.

**After all this preparation, how can the doctors be sure that
treatment is identical each day?**

When the doctor is satisfied with the treatment plan, the area to
be treated will be marked out on your body using an indelible
pen. These marks must not be removed until treatment is
finished. Sometimes a tiny ink spot the size of a pin head is
tattooed on the skin as a reference point. This will be permanent
but should be almost invisible to anyone not looking for it.

**I'm going to be having treatment to part of my face and neck.
I won't have to walk around with marks that everyone can
see, will I?**

No. Anyone who is going to have radiotherapy to the head or neck area will have an extra step in the planning procedure. A plastic shell or **mould** will be made. This serves two purposes: it helps you to keep your head very still during the treatment sessions and the marks which outline the treatment field can be drawn on the shell and not on you.

How is a mould made?

You will given an appointment to attend the mould room. Here specially trained technicians will position you on a couch and a quick-setting cream will be applied to your skin over the proposed treatment area. This is lifted off as soon as it has set and your individual plastic shell is made from this impression of your face.

If you have a beard or moustache you may be asked to shave it off before the mould is made so that the shell will fit closely to your skin.

This sounds quite unpleasant – is it?

Most people find this procedure unpleasant and some find it a claustrophobic experience. The plus side is that it is over very quickly and it does mean that your treatment can be given very accurately.

My young child is about to start radiotherapy. How will she be able to keep still through all this planning and then the treatment?

The doctors know how difficult it is for a child to keep still and also how upset they can be by all these new experiences. Your daughter may be given something to make her sleepy or even a short-acting, light general anaesthetic so that she is not unduly distressed by everything that is happening. In addition, you may be able to be with her throughout most of these procedures, except during the treatment itself, because it is important you are not exposed to radiation. Often the staff will spend time getting to know your child and will try to help her settle down.

What's it like having radiotherapy? You're left on your own, aren't you?

When you first attend for your radiotherapy treatment it can be quite frightening because you are on your own in a big room while the treatment is given. But you are not alone.

The radiographers, who supervise your therapy, will position you carefully on the treatment couch. When you are in the correct position, they will ask you to remain very still although, obviously, you can breathe and swallow normally. They will leave the room and switch on the radiotherapy machine. For a very short time you will be on your own, but the radiographers will be able to see you all the time either through a window or on a closed circuit television. You can talk to them if necessary and they to you by a system of microphones.

As soon as the treatment time is finished, the radiographers will return. If you have to have treatment from more than one angle, they will reposition you and leave again. The radiographers work with radiotherapy daily and it is important that they are not exposed to unnecessary radiation. This is why they cannot stay with you.

As treatment progresses you will get used to this procedure and probably wonder what you were so worried about. If you have any questions or concerns, talk to the radiographers who will advise you. They understand that this is a frightening experience for most people.

Will I get radiation sickness?

No. Radiation sickness is a term that is used to describe a whole series of symptoms which people experience when they have been exposed to large amounts of radiation after major nuclear accidents, such as the Chernobyl disaster.

You may feel nauseated or sick during some of the time you have radiotherapy but this is a specific side effect, not radiation sickness. It depends very much on the area of your body which is being irradiated.

Will my hair fall out?

Not necessarily. Hair is only lost from the part of the body which is being treated. If your axilla (armpit) is in the radiotherapy field you will lose hair there; if your chest is in the field you will lose any hair in that area; if your head is being treated you will lose hair from there. But you will not, for example, lose hair from your head if your chest is being treated. Hair usually grows again after treatment has finished.

Radiotherapy causes sore skin, doesn't it?

Sometimes your skin may become sore, but often it does not. Modern machines use what are called 'skin-sparing techniques'. The radiotherapy burns that people once talked about are rarely seen now. Always follow the advice you are given by the radiographers regarding care of your skin. If you do develop a skin reaction it is usually similar to a mild sunburn.

What other kind of side effects am I likely to experience during radiotherapy?

Some people experience no problems at all during radiotherapy and others, although they feel tired, have few side effects. Many people continue their normal social activities and work throughout their treatment. Other people may feel unwell before they start radiotherapy because of their illness, a recent operation or other treatment. In this situation radiation treatment may make existing symptoms worse.

Side effects are specific to the individual and to the area of the body which is being treated. Any side effects are usually temporary. Ask your doctor and the radiographers about what to expect in your case. Tell them if you experience any problems or unusual effects. There may be medication or other measures which can help you cope with side effects of treatment, for example if you do feel sick or suffer from diarrhoea.

Will I see the doctor during my course of radiotherapy?

Yes, you will probably see the doctor each week. You will also have regular blood tests to check your progress and you may have other investigations repeated during this time. You may have to go back to the simulator for adjustments to be made to your treatment plan. This is not unusual and does not mean that something is wrong.

If you are worried about anything during treatment, take the opportunity to discuss it with your doctor during your weekly consultation. Some people feel a bit low during radiotherapy and talking about this often helps.

Is there anything that I shouldn't do during radiation treatment?

You will be told if there is anything specific you should or shouldn't do, but here is a list of general points.

Do look after yourself, eat well and drink plenty of fluids. If you have problems with eating or lose your appetite, please mention this to the staff. There are lots of suggestions which can be offered to help with this and expert advice can be provided by a dietitian.

Do make sure you get plenty of rest. You might be able to carry on as usual but, on the other hand, you may find you can only work part-time or you may need help with shopping or housework.

Do wear clothes in which you feel comfortable. If you have treatment marks on your skin you might prefer to wear older clothes so new things are not marked by the ink. Loose-fitting underwear and clothes are best, as they will not rub on the treatment area and cause the skin to become sore.

Do take notice of the advice on skin care which will be given to you by the radiographers. The ink marks must not be washed off but you will normally be able to splash tepid water onto your skin and gently pat it dry to keep yourself feeling clean. You should not use soap, deodorants or perfume on an area within the treatment field but baby talcum powder is usually all right. Men should shave with an electric razor if the face or neck area is being treated to prevent irritation from soaps or creams.

Do keep your treatment area out of the sun or cold winds and don't use hot water bottles or ice packs. Although skin reactions are much less common now, your skin will be more sensitive.

Do ask if you are unsure about anything or have any specific concerns related to your personal treatment or side effects.

I've been told I'm to have Selectron treatment. What is it?

Selectron treatment is a type of internal radiotherapy frequently used to treat gynaecological cancers such as cancer of the cervix. It is given using a special machine which automatically places radioactive sources inside special tubes which have been inserted by the doctor into your vagina and/or uterus (womb). Treatment may be given at a low dose-rate over several hours in hospital, or a high dose-rate over a few minutes as an out-patient. Your treatment will be planned individually for you, just as carefully as external radiotherapy.

Ask your doctor for details of the treatment planned for you.

Chemotherapy

When someone has chemotherapy, are the drugs that are injected radioactive?

No. Chemotherapy and radiotherapy are completely different treatments.

What is chemotherapy?

Chemotherapy is treatment with drugs. They are called **cytotoxic** drugs, which literally means cell poisons. This form of therapy may be given to destroy or control cancer cells which are known to be present and are causing symptoms. It may also be given when the doctors know there is a high chance of cancer cells being present in the body even if they can't be detected at this moment.

What's the difference between chemotherapy and radiotherapy?

Radiotherapy is a local treatment. In other words it can only kill cancer cells within the field of the radiation beam. Chemotherapy is a systemic (whole body) treatment. The cytotoxic drugs circulate around the whole body in the bloodstream and can destroy cancer cells in different parts of the body.

Why do some people have radiotherapy and others have chemotherapy?

One reason is that some cancers are more sensitive to one treatment than to the other, that is one particular therapy is more effective in killing one particular type of cancer cell. The doctors will also know if a cancer is confined to just one area or has spread or if it is likely to spread which will indicate whether a local or systemic treatment is needed. Even people with the same cancer will have different treatments, based on the information available about their individual cases.

Increasingly surgery, radiotherapy, chemotherapy and other treatments are used together to achieve the best possible chance of cure or control. This is called adjuvant therapy.

How do the drugs work?

Cytotoxic drugs destroy cancer cells by interfering with their ability to grow and divide. Scientists now know exactly how some of the drugs work but in one or two cases their action is less clear. We don't know how they work, just that they do!

How is chemotherapy given?

The most common method of administration is an injection into a vein using a syringe or through an infusion ('drip'). Drugs may also be given as tablets or capsules and, occasionally, by injection into a muscle or under the skin.

There are other methods of giving chemotherapy, such as an injection into a body cavity like the chest, but these are less common. If drugs are to be given in a special way like this, the procedure and the reason for it will be explained.

Are there lots of different chemotherapy drugs?

Yes. There are over 30 cytotoxic drugs used to treat cancer. Scientists are working all the time to find new agents which are either more effective or have fewer side effects than existing drugs.

One friend of mine had chemotherapy and had to go into hospital but another had treatment as an out-patient. Is one treatment stronger than the other?

No. There are different ways of administering the drugs. Some can be given over a few minutes but others must be given over a number of hours. Often extra fluids and drugs need to be given together with the chemotherapy. A hospital stay of 24–48 hours may be necessary.

There may be other reasons why your friend was admitted to hospital. Perhaps she was unwell before her chemotherapy was started or maybe the expected side effects could be better prevented or controlled in hospital.

Do you just have one drug at a time?

Not necessarily. A person may have one drug, several drugs together or different drugs at different times. Your individual treatment will be prescribed and explained by your doctor.

Is there a particular name for doctors who specialise in drug treatment?

Yes, they are called **medical oncologists**.

Is chemotherapy given as a course of treatment similar to radiotherapy?

Yes, but whereas radiotherapy is planned over a few weeks, chemotherapy usually continues for several months.

Does this mean I'm having treatment all the time?

No, although this will depend on the specific treatment or **regime** chosen for you. Usually each course of treatment is followed by a 'rest' period. This rest period is often longer than the treatment time and its purpose is to allow your body to recover from the effects of the drugs. For example, you may have an injection one week, another the following week and then three weeks off treatment.

Won't the cancer cells continue growing during the rest period?

This is unlikely. The cytotoxic effect of the drugs carries on after the treatment days. Because cancer cells do not recover as quickly as normal cells, the repeated treatments gradually reduce the number of cancer cells which are, or may be, present in your body.

How long is a course of chemotherapy?

The length of treatment usually depends on how well your disease responds to the drugs. Your doctor will be constantly checking this using blood tests, x-rays, scans and other investigations. Most people receive chemotherapy for about six months.

My doctor says my chemotherapy is an 'insurance policy'. How does he know it's working?

When a person has adjuvant therapy, as you describe, there is no immediate way of knowing if it is working because there is no disease to assess. Your doctor will have considered two things: the results of research which show that chemotherapy can reduce the risk of the cancer coming back and also, from that research, how long chemotherapy needs to be given to people in similar circumstances to yours in order to be most effective.

My cancer didn't disappear with the first combination of drugs the doctor recommended. Can I have more treatment?

The answer to this is usually yes. The doctors now know which drugs work with different types of cancer and they can put these together in different combinations until the best one is found for you. It may be necessary to try one or two regimes before the most effective combination is discovered.

You hear stories about how awful chemotherapy is. Are there lots of side effects?

Not always. Some people experience few side effects during chemotherapy and are able to continue with their normal activities. For others, chemotherapy is a miserable experience and the effect on their lives is considerable.

Any side effects which occur depend on which of the many drugs are prescribed for you. In addition each person reacts in an individual way to chemotherapy. It is not always helpful to listen to other people's experiences of chemotherapy as effects can vary so much. Two people receiving the same combination of drugs may feel completely different during their courses of treatment.

Why do side effects occur?

Cytotoxic drugs destroy cells which are constantly dividing – a characteristic of cancer cells. But normal, healthy cells also grow and divide to repair body tissues, and so these cells will be damaged too. It is this damage which causes side effects. Fortunately normal cells recover quickly so side effects of treatment are usually temporary.

Are side effects inevitable?

It is impossible to say because so much depends on the drug or drugs you are to receive. The doctors and nurses will be able to tell you what to expect and also offer advice on how to cope with any side effects. Some of the more common side effects are dealt with in the following questions.

I've been told that once I start treatment I will have to have regular blood tests. Why is this necessary?

One of the side effects of chemotherapy is 'bone marrow depression'. Your bone marrow is the factory where blood cells are made and, because this is a continuous process, these cells are frequently affected by cytotoxic drugs. By examining the number of blood cells at regular intervals during treatment, the doctors can make sure that the bone marrow is not being affected too much by the drugs.

What would happen if the numbers of blood cells being made was reduced?

If your blood cells or **blood count** was low, the doctor would either adjust the dose of your drugs or lengthen your rest period between treatments. Although it is worrying and frustrating when this happens, it is not unusual. It is much safer to delay treatment by about a week than to give the drugs before your 'count' has recovered.

What is counted when a blood sample is examined?

There are three types of blood cells which are each separately measured in your blood count:
(i)   white blood cells which help you to fight infection;
(ii)   platelets which help the blood to clot, preventing bleeding and bruising; and
(iii) red blood cells which carry oxygen to the tissues of the body.

If my blood count falls, what effect will it have on me?

Very often you will not notice anything unusual. Sometimes people say that they feel a bit depressed and tired when their count is at its lowest about 10-14 days after treatment. However, if your count has dropped, or is expected to, you may be told to look out for certain signs or symptoms which should be reported to your doctor.

What kind of things might indicate that my blood count is low?

When your white cells are low, you will be more likely to develop an infection. You should contact your doctor if you have a sore throat or start running a high temperature, or if you notice anything else that might mean you have an infection, such as a burning sensation when you pass urine.

A drop in your platelet count will mean you may bruise more easily. You might notice that your gums bleed when you brush your teeth, or you might have a nosebleed.

If your red blood cells are affected, you will become anaemic and may feel tired or short of breath.

It is very important that you report anything unusual for you to the doctor straight away, even if it seems trivial. You may need a course of antibiotics to fight an infection or a transfusion of blood or platelets to increase the numbers of these cells in the blood.

New drugs called **colony stimulating factors** are now available, which can help to increase your white cell count. You may be given one of these drugs immediately after your treatment to reduce the likelihood of you developing an infection or of your chemotherapy dose having to be adjusted.

If I need a blood transfusion, is there a risk of catching AIDS?

All donor blood is tested for the HIV virus, which causes AIDS, and people in known high-risk groups are discouraged from giving blood. In addition, blood products are heat treated to destroy the virus. The risk of transfer of the disease in this way is very small indeed.

My child is having chemotherapy for leukaemia. Surely if all the abnormal and the normal blood cells are destroyed he might die?

At the present time, the abnormal cells in your child's bone marrow are preventing normal blood cells from growing. The cytotoxic drugs will destroy the leukaemic cells and allow the normal cells to increase in number. The drugs used at this stage of treatment are specially chosen so that the normal blood cells are damaged as little as possible.

Will I feel sick?

You may feel nauseated, or even vomit, following your chemotherapy but this is not a side effect of every drug. To a large extent the doctors can predict which drugs will cause a greater reaction in the majority of people. You will be given anti-emetic (anti-sickness) drugs to take during, and immediately after, your treatment to reduce any nausea or vomiting. You may be admitted to hospital if it is thought you will be sick in order that more effective medications can be given to you.

Some newer anti-emetic drugs can prevent or greatly reduce nausea and vomiting. In addition the staff caring for you may be able to offer other suggestions to reduce sickness, such as changes in eating patterns and learning relaxation techniques.

If one anti-sickness drug doesn't work, can I try another?

Yes. Tell the doctor or nurse before your next treatment. There are several drugs which can be prescribed.

Will my hair fall out?

This depends on the drug or combination of drugs you are receiving. It is not a side effect of every chemotherapy regime – some cytotoxic drugs always cause hair loss and some never do. Often the hair will become thinner or lose its body. No-one but you may notice this.

In order to keep your hair in good condition treat it gently. Avoid having it coloured or permed and don't use a hot hair dryer or heated rollers. Anything which can damage your hair (such as brushing it too hard or plaiting it) should also be avoided. Always ask for advice if you are in any doubt about what you should or should not do.

Sometimes a procedure called 'scalp cooling', which restricts blood flow to the hair roots at the time of the injection, may prevent hair loss. It cannot be used for every drug, or every person.

Will my hair grow back?

Hair loss is always temporary and the hair grows back in the months after treatment. Occasionally the hair starts to regrow before the end of a course of chemotherapy.

If I'm going to lose my hair, how soon will it happen and what can I do about it?

First of all, if it is predicted you will lose your hair, arrangements can be made for you to obtain a wig before your treatment starts. The time before the hair begins to fall out varies from a few days to a few weeks. You will probably notice more hair in your brush or comb and, most upsetting of all, hair on your pillow in the mornings. Wearing a hairnet or turban overnight is a good idea. Some people, particularly men, prefer to shave their heads as soon as the hair starts coming out.

If you don't want to wear a wig all or even part of the time a cap, hat or attractive scarf is an alternative. Protect your scalp from the cold and the sun by using some form of covering or a sunblock cream. If your scalp becomes dry, use a gentle moisturiser.

Will I lose my body hair?

Some drugs do cause loss of body hair. Ask if this is expected in your case.

When my hair grows back will it be the same as before I lost it?

Not always. Sometimes the hair grows back a different colour. It may be curly instead of straight or vice versa. It is not possible to predict in advance whether this will happen to you.

My chemotherapy is in tablet form. Will these make me feel sick?

Possibly: you may find that taking the tablets at night will solve this problem. Check with your doctor if you can do this.

Is having chemotherapy painful?

Chemotherapy is no more painful than having an injection or a blood test. During a course of treatment your veins may become sensitive or sore and you should tell your doctor or nurse if this happens so that these areas can be avoided.

My child is about to start chemotherapy and this will be given through a Hickman line. What is a Hickman line?

A Hickman line is a special catheter (tube) which is inserted into a large vein, through the chest wall. It can be left in place for many months. Drugs and fluids can be given through the catheter and blood samples can also be taken from it. It removes the need for repeated injections into veins in the arm or hand. It is not limited to children: some adults will also have a Hickman catheter.

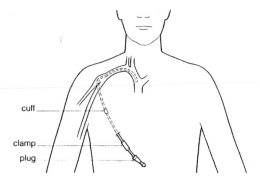

cuff

clamp

plug

Figure 2: Hickman catheter (reproduced by kind permission of the Royal Marsden Hospital)

Why do some people have a Hickman catheter and others don't?

Many people simply don't need one, for example if their chemotherapy is only for a short time or involves only an occasional injection. However, if treatment is going to continue for many months and extra fluids or other drugs are required, the doctors may decide that it is better to put in a Hickman line (central venous catheter).

Can I eat and drink normally during chemotherapy?

Yes. You may find you lose your appetite for a few days after your treatment but when it returns to normal you can eat your usual foods. Try to drink about twice as much as normal while you are having chemotherapy. Generally, it will be all right to have an occasional alcoholic drink. You will be told if you should not drink alcohol or if there are any foods you should avoid.

If you have any problems with eating tell your doctor or nurse. They may be able to offer some suggestions or ask the dietitian to advise you.

My periods have stopped since I started chemotherapy. Is this normal?

It is not unusual for your periods to become irregular or stop during chemotherapy. This is temporary and does not mean you cannot conceive. It is not advisable for you to become pregnant during or immediately after chemotherapy, so you must use an effective form of contraception throughout treatment. The same advice applies during and after radiotherapy.

Can I take the contraceptive pill?

It is best to check with your doctor about this. She or he will be able to advise you on alternative contraceptive methods if continuing with the pill is not recommended.

If I have chemotherapy will I become sterile?

In men sterility can occur, but it is not a side effect of many drugs. It is usually temporary. If permanent sterility is anticipated, you will be offered an opportunity to 'bank' sperm before starting treatment. Once again, contraception should be used during and after chemotherapy. If you wish to father a child later discuss this with your doctor.

Does chemotherapy make you impotent?

Sexual performance is not usually affected by the drugs, but any physical illness or anxiety about treatment can cause temporary sexual difficulties.

My daughter is getting married soon and the dates coincide with my treatment. Can I change the day of my injection?

Usually the doctors are quite willing to change treatment dates by a few days to fit in with special occasions like a wedding, or so you can have a short holiday. Ask your doctor if it's possible to reorganise your dates.

Will I see the doctor regularly during treatment?

Yes: you will see the doctor every time you come into hospital for chemotherapy and when you start each course of treatment as an out-patient. She or he will ask for regular tests, like x-rays or scans, to check your general health and how the chemotherapy is affecting you.

The doctor will want to know how you feel. Talk about

anything unusual you may have experienced, whether it was expected or not. And also use this time to discuss any worries you may have and to ask questions. Don't worry if a physical change or a concern that you have seems trivial – it is always best to check. Always ask the doctor before taking other medicines and, if you wish to try a complementary therapy, find out if there is any reason why you should not use it at this time.

Hormone Therapy

Is hormone therapy a type of chemotherapy?

Hormone therapy is treatment with medicines so it could possibly be thought of as a type of chemotherapy, but hormones don't work in the same way as cytotoxic drugs.

What are hormones?

Hormones are natural substances which occur in all our bodies and affect or control the function of certain of our organs or systems. For example, a woman's menstrual cycle (her periods) is controlled by hormones called oestrogen and progesterone. Testosterone is the hormone which causes a boy's voice to deepen and his body hair to grow during adolescence.

How can hormones be used to treat cancer?

Certain cancers are know to be affected by the level of hormones in the body, and hormone therapy takes advantage of this fact. When doctors recommend hormone therapy it usually does one of three things. The level of a particular hormone may be reduced, the action of a hormone may be 'blocked' (its effect is stopped), or a hormone level may be increased. Doctors call this hormonal manipulation (change).

When are hormones used to treat cancer?

Hormones are a systemic treatment, that is a treatment which can reach all parts of the body. They may be used to treat or control disease which is known to be present and is causing symptoms, but they may also be used when there is a high chance of cancer cells being present although these cannot be detected. Hormone therapy may also be used in addition to surgery, radiotherapy or chemotherapy in the treatment of cancer, to achieve the best possible chance of cure or control. This is called adjuvant therapy.

Are steroids hormones?

Yes. Steroids are normally produced by the body and affect a number of its functions. We often hear about steroids being abused by people involved in sports who want to build up their muscles and achieve false levels of fitness. When steroids are given as treatment they are carefully controlled.

What types of cancer can be treated by hormone therapy?

The main types of cancer treated by hormones are certain tumours of the breast, prostate, thyroid and uterus (womb). Leukaemia and lymphomas (cancers of the lymphatic system) such as Hodgkin's disease can also be treated with hormones.

How do hormones work?

Most hormone therapy works by changing the balance of hormones in the body and this affects the cancer. Steroids also have a cytotoxic action, like the drugs used in chemotherapy.

How are hormones given?

The most common method of giving hormones is by mouth as tablets. Some hormones are injected, usually into a muscle.

How long is a course of hormone therapy?

Hormone therapy is usually given over a number of months or years. Obviously, if a cancer is present and does not respond to therapy, the treatment will be stopped and a different treatment started in its place. If hormones are given as adjuvant therapy, as in the case of breast cancer, they will be given for a set period of time, usually two years. Research has shown that the effect of this treatment can be seen as increased cure and survival 10 years on.

I'm taking hormone replacement therapy. Is this the same as hormone therapy?

Hormone replacement therapy (HRT) is used to treat symptoms which occur at the time of the menopause. Hormone therapy is used to treat some cancers. Although both treatments use hormones, different ones will be given and the purpose of treatment is different.

If you have had cancer you may receive HRT if your treatment has caused an early menopause, for example if your ovaries have been removed.

Are there any side effects from hormone therapy?

Yes, but these will vary depending on which hormone you are taking. If your doctor recommends hormone therapy, ask what effects and side effects you should expect.

Is Tamoxifen a hormone?

Yes. Tamoxifen is an anti-oestrogen drug which has been shown to be very effective in the treatment of breast cancer. It is a hormone which also has few side effects. If it is prescribed for you, ask about these and, as with any treatment, report back to your doctor anything unusual which you experience during therapy. Any side effects will cease at the end of treatment.

Can Tamoxifen prevent breast cancer?

No-one knows at the present time. Because of the success of Tamoxifen in the treatment of breast cancer, doctors are doing research to discover if the risk can be reduced in women with a family history of the disease. It will be several years before the results of this research are available.

Does hormone therapy for prostate cancer cause impotence?

Yes, because the action of the male hormone testosterone is blocked. Impotence is usually only for the duration of treatment.

People who take steroids put on weight and get puffy faces, don't they?

Steroids can cause more water to be held in the body, leading to weight gain and a puffy face. Steroids also improve the appetite and eating more than usual will cause you to put on weight too. The effects of steroid therapy gradually disappear after treatment finishes.

Biological therapies

What are biological therapies?

They are a new group of treatments which are natural substances made by the immune system (the body's defence system). There are two main types: **cytokines**, which are generally used in the treatment of particular cancers and **colony stimulating factors**, which are used to reduce the side effects of chemotherapy.

How do biological therapies work?

Biological therapy agents act as on/off switches on the cells of the immune (defence) system. They control cell growth, increase normal activity against cancer cells or raise the production of antibodies (specific types of proteins in the blood) to fight cancer cells. Colony stimulating factors, for example, increase the number of white blood cells (the cells which help you fight infections) being produced during chemotherapy.

I've heard of interferon – is that a biological therapy?

Yes – **interferon** (which has received a great deal of publicity) is a cytokine, as are substances called **interleukins**.

The colony stimulating factors include **G-CSF** (granulocyte colony stimulating factor) and **GM-CSF** (granulocyte macrophage colony stimulating factor). Each of these agents stimulates a different type of white blood cell.

When are cytokines used?

All cytokines have an effect throughout the body so they are mainly used when disease is widespread. Most of these substances are still being tested in clinical trials (research studies) and few are as yet used as standard treatment for cancer. Occasionally cytokines are used on their own but more often they are combined with chemotherapy.

Which cancers may be treated with cytokines?

At the present time, very few. Interferon is used to treat a form of leukaemia called hairy cell leukaemia. Interleukin-2 is used for people with renal (kidney) cancer and for malignant melanoma, a form of skin cancer.

Why are colony stimulating factors used?

These agents can be used to help your body recover from the effects of treatment. G-CSF and GM-CSF increase the number of white blood cells being produced during chemotherapy. This means that you might be able to have chemotherapy more frequently or at higher doses than usual. The rest periods between treatments might not have to be lengthened because your white blood count becomes low (which increases your chance of having an infection). Your overall time on treatment might not have to be changed from what was originally proposed, for example six months.

How are biological therapies given?

All therapy is given by injection, sometimes into a vein but usually under the skin. People are often taught to give their own injections because treatment continues for a long time. Admission to hospital may be necessary at the beginning of your treatment but after that you can continue it as an out-patient.

How long is treatment given for?

Cytokine treatment is given in long cycles, for example a daily injection for six weeks followed by a rest period before the next cycle is started. Therapy continues for months rather than weeks because the effect on the cancer is not seen straight away. It may be quite a time before the doctor can tell you if the treatment is working to control your disease.

Treatment with colony stimulating factors usually lasts for 7–10 days; it will be given after each course of chemotherapy.

Clinical trials

If the treatment for my cancer doesn't work or my cancer comes back after the first treatment I have, what happens then?

Your doctor will probably recommend another course of therapy. This may be a second operation, another course of radiotherapy or more chemotherapy. She or he may also want to try a new treatment like one of the biological therapies or a new approach to treatment which is currently being studied in a clinical trial.

What is a clinical trial?

A clinical trial is a scientific study of a new investigation or treatment for cancer or a different way of giving care or relieving symptoms. A trial may also be used to compare a new treatment with the best standard treatment currently available. Two methods of giving the same treatment may be tested against each other. Much of what is now accepted as standard treatment has been tested in this way in previous years. Doctors rely on the results of clinical trials when they give you advice on treatment now.

How will I know if I'm in a clinical trial?

Your doctor should tell you at the very beginning that the treatment option being recommended for you is a clinical trial or a research study. One of the questions you might like to ask your doctor is 'Is this a trial?' or 'Is this a research project?'

If any of the other staff caring for you, such as the nurses, are conducting a study of any kind you should also be informed.

Do I have to give my permission before I can be entered into a trial?

Yes. Your doctor or other staff have to gain your consent before they can do anything to you. You sign a consent form before an operation and many hospitals now ask for your written consent before some investigations, or before a course of radiotherapy or chemotherapy. You must agree to what the doctors propose before they can proceed. This is even more important if you are being asked to enter a research project.

What should I know about the research?

There are several things you should be told, for example what the trial involves, what benefits you may expect from it, what side effects might occur, and what it means to you in the way of extra tests, extra visits to hospital and so on.

You should be given some written information and allowed time to think about your decision. You may find there are more questions you want to ask in order to understand what is planned. You should not give your consent until you are completely happy about the project.

What if I say no?

You have the right to say yes or no to any treatment which is suggested for you. If you do not wish to take part in a trial you should say so. Your doctor will then discuss with you any other treatments which are available.

Can I change my mind?

Yes. If you decide later that you would like to take part in the research study, you can discuss this with your doctor. Similarly, if you have agreed to enter the trial, you may withdraw at any time without giving a reason. You can then discuss alternative treatment with your doctor.

Are there different types of trials?

Yes. There are many different ways in which trials are organised and several methods of analyzing statistics or information. A booklet **Clinical Trials** is available: details are given in Appendix II.

Have clinical trials really been of benefit to people with cancer?

Yes, although until recently the term 'research' was used instead, so many people think these trials are new. 'Research' and 'clinical trials' are really the same thing.

Many advances have been made in the diagnosis of cancer, in surgical and radiotherapy techniques and in ways of caring for people with cancer. In addition, the majority of drugs now used have been developed and introduced into everyday therapy in this way. Improvements in both cures and survival rates for many malignancies in children and adults have come about through research. These include new techniques of giving radiation therapy, high dose chemotherapy, bone marrow transplants and methods of drug administration that are associated with fewer side effects.

Research continues into better ways of preventing, detecting and treating cancer, and of caring for people with cancer.

How do I find out if there is a trial being run somewhere else which might benefit me?

First of all, ask your doctor who may know of research being carried out in a regional oncology centre or specialist hospital. Secondly, you might like to ring another hospital direct particularly if you have seen something about a trial in a newspaper or on television. And finally, you might be able to find out from one of the cancer information services whose addresses are listed in Appendix I.

Remember, even if a new treatment is being tried for people with the same cancer as you, **you** might not be 'eligible' for the trial.

What does 'eligible' mean?

When the doctors design a clinical trial, they have to lay down very strict guidelines as to who is included in the research, for example based on the stage of your disease. If you don't fit within these guidelines you will not be able to receive the new treatment.

Can't I get the new treatment if I'm able to pay for it?

No, offering to pay will make no difference if a clinical trial is being used to test or evaluate a new treatment.

If I go as a private patient from the start of my treatment, will I get better care and a better range of treatment choices?

Not necessarily. You might be able to recover from an operation in a single room rather than a ward, or arrange for more convenient appointment times but generally you will get equally good treatment and care within the NHS. In regional centres you might even have access to a wider range of services.

If I'm not satisfied with my treatment can I obtain a second opinion?

Yes. Discuss this with your hospital doctor. You will need a letter of referral to another specialist. If your hospital doctor is unhappy about your request, you can discuss this with your family doctor who is also able to refer you on for another opinion.

Most doctors are sympathetic in this situation. They understand that when faced with a diagnosis of cancer everyone wants to have the best treatment for themselves or their family.

If my doctor says that nothing more can be done, is this true?

It may be that nothing more can be offered from the point of view of standard treatment, but that the treatment offered within a clinical trial might mean control of the disease is possible. Alternatively the doctor may mean that no more active standard or clinical trial treatment is available to control the cancer.

It **does not** mean that nothing more can be done for you. A great deal can be offered to relieve symptoms and care for you. This is called palliative care and is covered in Chapter 7.

I don't want any more treatment. Can I refuse what the doctor offers?

Yes. You can refuse any treatment, in the same way you can agree to therapy. The decision is yours. Your doctor will respect your wishes. This is also one of the times when some people decide to explore different complementary therapies.

4
Complementary therapies

Introduction

This chapter answers some of the most common questions which people who have cancer ask about the use of complementary therapies, and explains some of the therapies in a little more detail. Please remember that there is no scientific evidence to show that any of the therapies listed can either cure cancer or control it. Having said that, many people find that using them helps them to improve their 'quality of life', that is their physical, emotional and psychological well-being.

You can get more information about the therapies mentioned in this chapter by contacting the relevant national association or organisation - addresses are listed in Appendix I.

What are complementary therapies?

Complementary therapies are, as the name suggests, treatments or therapies that may complement or supplement the 'conventional' medical treatments already described in Chapter 3. You might, for example, find one or more of these therapies useful in reducing the amount of stress you feel, or in helping you to relax during or after your treatment. They are also sometimes referred to as 'supportive' therapies.

Many complementary therapies require you to take an active part: this can enable you to feel as though you are doing something to help yourself. For some people, using one or more complementary therapies also brings a sense of taking control, as it is a part of their treatment which they have chosen to use rather than had prescribed for them.

What's the difference between complementary therapies and alternative therapies?

Complementary therapies used to be referred to as alternative therapies. This implied that they should be used instead of 'conventional' medical treatments. The change in name reflects a change in attitude: they are now seen as additional, rather than separate, options.

Are there many to choose from?

Dozens! But those which may be helpful for people who have cancer are described in this chapter.

Do complementary therapies work?

That's a question that doesn't have a direct answer. Some people swear by one method and may choose to use it as their sole treatment for cancer. Others try one or more therapies during and after they have had radiotherapy or chemotherapy. Not everyone will find that they benefit from using complementary techniques, but for many people the option to at least try is all important.

It is perhaps worth mentioning that not everyone wants to use complementary therapies. No-one should be pushed into trying something they are not sure about just because a relative or friend is convinced it would be helpful.

How do they help?

Many complementary therapies are concerned with taking an **holistic** approach to a person. 'Holistic' means that you are seen as a whole person in terms of your physical body, your mind and your spirit. Physical symptoms you might be experiencing from your cancer or your treatment are taken into account together with your feelings and emotions. So it's not simply a question having treatment given to a particular part of you. Rather it involves letting a practitioner know how you are feeling in a broader sense, in order that you can work together to face the cancer and any treatment and side effects you might experience. The therapies are unlikely completely to remove the side effects of some treatments, but you might find you can use them to help to reduce those you do have.

Therapies which focus on your emotional and psychological well-being may be aimed at stimulating your immune system by helping you to relax and so reduce any stress or tension you might have. These therapies can provide you with a role to play in your own treatment and can encourage you to develop a positive outlook or attitude. Feeling as though you are doing something to help yourself can give you a tremendous boost.

Can I use complementary therapies instead of having other hospital treatments?

Yes, if you wish to. You can decide whether or not to have any type of treatment that is offered to you, 'conventional' or complementary.

Will my doctor refuse to treat me if I use complementary therapies?

No doctor should refuse to treat a person who wishes to use complementary therapies alongside hospital treatment, as long as the therapies used are not likely to interfere with the hospital treatment or to make any side effects worse. The majority of cancer specialists now accept the idea of their patients using therapies that are concerned with providing emotional and psychological support. They may, however, be less keen on other therapies. If you find this to be so you should ask why, in case there are valid medical reasons against your choice.

How do I choose a therapy which will be right for me?

There are many complementary therapies and therapists, and choosing between them can be very difficult. You could talk to others who have used them, contact some of the organisations listed in Appendix I to find out more information about them, visit centres where different therapies are practised, read books about them ... and then try one or more that appeal to you.

Should the particular cancer I have influence my decision?

Yes, it should, as some therapies might not be helpful in certain cases. For example, a deep massage might not be helpful if you have cancer that has spread to several organs or bones, whereas a gentle massage might be relaxing and help you to feel good.

You should tell the practitioner what cancer you have and what other treatment you are having or have had, even if it is some time ago. If you are still having treatment or regular check ups at a hospital, you might also want to ask the opinion of one of the health professionals there.

Should the hospital treatment I'm having affect my choice of complementary therapy?

Yes, it should. Some hospital treatments cause side effects that might be made worse if a particular therapy is being used at the same time. For example, if you are having radiotherapy treatment that includes your bladder or bowels you are quite likely to experience diarrhoea as your treatment progresses. The staff in the radiotherapy department should give you some suggestions about the type of diet you should eat to try to reduce this side effect. If you decide instead to follow a particular complementary diet that recommends eating a lot of fresh fruit and vegetables you may find your symptoms of diarrhoea are made worse. If you wish to follow this particular complementary diet you might be better advised to wait until after the radiotherapy and its side effects have finished.

How do I know if a therapist would be suitable to work with people who have cancer?

A qualified therapist should not take you on as a client without first knowing all the relevant facts about you. If you are not asked directly you should tell the therapist about the cancer and any treatment you have had. If she or he then feels that the therapy might be unsuitable for someone who has cancer, it is unlikely that they will suggest you start to work with them. A good practitioner should advise you against a therapy that might adversely affect your cancer.

Do all therapists have recognised qualifications?

Many types of complementary therapies require practitioners to belong to a national association. The association should be concerned with training and qualifications, and should not permit any member to practise if they have not satisfied some specific criteria or are not suitably qualified.

Before you choose a therapy you should check out these facts by contacting the relevant association as well as asking the practitioner. In this way you should be able to avoid the charlatans as well as ensuring that you find a trained therapist.

Is using a complementary therapy expensive?

Very few therapies are available on the NHS and those that are may not be widely available. Many therapies involve a course of treatment lasting for several sessions and this could prove costly. Before you decide to embark on a course of treatment, you should ask exactly how many times you will be expected to attend, how often and how much it will cost.

Do complementary therapies take up much time?

Some do and some don't. Once you have learned how to use relaxation techniques you may find you can take a few minutes out relaxing whenever you like. On the other hand counselling may require you to travel to the counsellor, have the session and travel back again, perhaps at a regular time each week for a number of weeks.

What if I don't have the willpower to keep using a particular therapy?

Many people worry that if they start to use one therapy or another they will be committing themselves to having to continue for a long time, and some of the therapies mentioned in this chapter do require a lot of willpower. But if you do not want to carry on (whatever your reasons) it is important for you to stop, or you will be left feeling tied to something that started out as a matter of choice.

But then how do you stop feeling that you've failed and have let everyone down?

Just as choosing to use a particular therapy should be a decision you make for yourself, so stopping its use is equally your decision. It is not a question of failing, rather it is a question of having tried something that is not right for you. No-one else can really know how you are feeling, so no-one else has the right to tell you to continue when you do not want to.

Sometimes people stop using a therapy because it is too expensive or because they can no longer give the time necessary. It can be very hard to reach such a decision without feeling guilty about stopping, particularly if relatives or friends had been eager for you to take up the therapy in the first place. Yet, once again, the decision belongs to you and no-one should attach blame or be angry about your choice.

Acupuncture

What is acupuncture?

Acupuncture is a type of medicine which has been practised for several thousand years. In China it is a standard form of medical treatment. The key principles behind it are:

(i)   we all have a vital energy called **Ch'i** flowing throughout our bodies along pathways called meridians;
(ii) if we are ill it is due to an imbalance in the body's Ch'i;
(iii) this means that at least one of our 12 meridians is blocked – the Ch'i is not able to flow and so symptoms of disease appear in the parts of the body corresponding to the meridians;
(iv) by inserting very fine special needles into certain points which lie along the meridians, energy can be diverted to areas where it is needed to treat the imbalance in Ch'i.

Can acupuncture be used to treat all cancers?

No, but it can be used to provide some pain relief or to treat nausea or muscle spasms.

How many sessions are needed to be effective?

This is hard to say. How long treatment will last and how often you will need it to maintain any beneficial effects will vary from person to person. It will also depend on why you are having it and how long you have had the symptoms that you wish to treat.

Is acupuncture available on the NHS?

Some acupuncturists do provide treatment on the NHS, working in hospitals or clinics.

Do acupuncturists have to be specially trained?

Yes, they do. Some acupuncturists are medically qualified doctors or dentists who have then been trained in acupuncture. Others may not have a medical background but have been trained as acupuncturists.

Art therapy

What is art therapy?

Art therapy is a way of communicating your feelings and thoughts without words. You draw or paint whatever comes to mind and you may then choose to discuss your picture with the art therapist. As you do so, you may find you become aware of things you hadn't previously realised or recognised.

Do you have to be able to draw in the first place?

No, definitely not! Art therapy isn't about creating works of art: it's about using paper and paints or crayons to express yourself without having to find words.

Is art therapy useful for people who have cancer?

Yes, it can be very useful, because it can help you to gain a greater understanding of yourself and of the cancer and treatment you are experiencing as well as helping you to express your feelings.

How many sessions do you have?

That depends on you and on the art therapist with whom you work. Some people start to use art therapy when they are diagnosed as having cancer and continue to use it throughout their treatment and beyond. Others may be introduced to it for the first time when they are terminally ill and may find it helps them to face dying. Some people find drawing helpful even if they don't always share their work with an art therapist.

Is it available on the NHS?

Art therapy is sometimes available in cancer treatment centres and hospices.

Are art therapists specially trained?

Yes, there are training courses which a person undertakes in order to practise as an art therapist. There are various approaches used in art therapy and the training differs for each of these. Some training in one or more psychological techniques will be included, so that interpretations of your paintings can be made with you.

Counselling

What is counselling?

Counselling is a process which involves the practitioner, or counsellor, listening carefully to what the person, or client, is saying about a particular situation or experience, and then responding in a way that enables the client to explore and to understand more clearly what she or he is feeling and thinking about the situation or experience. It is private and confidential.

Is counselling the same thing as giving advice?

No, it is not. Giving advice, directing you to take a particular course of action or passing judgement on something you have said or have done is not counselling. 'If I were you I'd ...' is an example of giving advice. 'What do you think you might find helpful ...?' is an example of using a counselling approach.

How can it help someone who has cancer?

It can provide a space and a place for someone who has cancer to talk about their feelings, or about events current and past as well as hopes and fears for the future.

There are different types of counselling which can be broadly split into those which focus on aspects of behaviour, those which are concerned with your past life and experiences, and those which concentrate on you as you are today. Different techniques suit different people, so if you try one type of counselling and it doesn't feel right you might want to try another type with another counsellor.

How many sessions are needed for it to be effective?

This varies from person to person and between different types of counselling. The first time you go to see a counsellor you should end the session by both agreeing to a 'contract'. This covers how many times you plan to meet, how much each session will cost, how long sessions will last and where they will take place. Although it is called a 'contract', it is not a legal agreement! 'Contract' is simply a word to describe whatever you and the counsellor have decided between you. You can, of course, change your 'contract' at any time, or give up your counselling sessions if you wish to do so.

Is counselling available on the NHS?

More and more cancer treatment centres employ counsellors who may be nurses or radiographers who should have had special counselling training. Local cancer support and self help groups may have counsellors in the group who will see people free of charge or for a small fee. Private counsellors will charge fees; some offer concessionary rates if you ask for them.

Do counsellors have to be specially trained?

If they are to practise as counsellors they should have completed a professional training course.

What is the difference between counselling and counselling skills?

Many people who provide support and a listening ear for people who have cancer have not been professionally trained as counsellors but have very good counselling skills. This means that they are able to listen to what the person is saying and to respond in a caring and empathic way. They will not enter into a 'contract' of the sort described above and usually provide their services for free.

Diets

Is there a special diet I should eat because I have cancer?

No, there isn't one special diet to follow. Everyone, whether they have cancer or not, is advised to eat a well balanced diet. For most people this means cutting down on the amount of fatty food they eat and having more fresh fruit and vegetables. This is a standard recommendation for general health, not a complementary therapy! Such a diet could be as helpful for the people you live with as it is for you.

Why do some people decide to follow a new diet when they have cancer?

Following a new diet can lead some people to feel that they are helping themselves in a positive way. For some people a change in their diet can lead to a change in their attitude towards themselves.

What sort of diets are there?

There are many different diets that people who have cancer might wish to try, and some of the better known ones are mentioned here.

It is always advisable to tell the health professionals who are involved in your hospital treatment if you are planning to change your usual diet during the time you are having treatment, as some diets may make expected side effects of treatment (for example diarrhoea) much worse. Hospital dietitians should be able to provide you with dietary advice specific for your needs during and immediately after treatment.

Some dietary therapies can require a lot of preparation and can be very time consuming and expensive. This could have a big impact on any other people who live with you, and you might wish to take this into account if you are choosing between several diets.

What is the Bristol Diet?

This is a diet that was first used at the **Bristol Cancer Help Centre** – the address is given in Appendix I. Originally it was based on a very strict vegan diet of raw vegetables. Animal products, salt and certain refined carbohydrates were not allowed, and very little fat or sugar was included.

Recently it has been adapted and is now less stringent. It is no longer called the Bristol Diet and each person is given individual attention to help them to use nutrition as a self-help tool. The diet now is a wholefood diet, offering vegetarian and vegan approaches as well as including some animal protein as appropriate.

Gerson Therapy involves a diet, doesn't it?

Yes, it does. Gerson Therapy views cancer as a chronic disease which upsets the body's metabolism, leading to tissue damage (especially in the liver) and to the immune system (the body's defence system) being less able to fight off infection. The therapy aims to help to make the body healthy by making the immune system function properly again.

The diet is one of fruit and vegetables which may be eaten raw, liquidised or steamed. Liver extracts and potassium supplements are also taken. Gerson Therapy involves using coffee or castor oil enemas to help to stimulate the liver to remove poisons from the body.

What is the Macrobiotic Diet?

This diet is based on eating foods which complement each other in terms of **Yin** and **Yang**. Yin and Yang are two opposing but complementary principles in Chinese philosophy. Yin, which comes from the Chinese word for dark, represents feminine, dark and negative principles. Yang, which comes from the Chinese word for light, represents masculine, light and positive principles. Illness is attributed to an imbalance of these two principles.

Yin foods include fruit, and sweet, sour or hot foods, while Yang foods include cereals and foods of animal origin. By adapting your dietary balance of Yin and Yang foods to counteract the imbalance you may restore your health. Salt intake is strictly controlled and processed foods are not eaten at all in this diet.

Many people are vegetarian, but what does this mean?

A vegetarian diet is one that does not include any meat products. Some vegetarians also avoid some or all of dairy products, eggs or fish. If they do not eat any of these animal products at all (for example using soya milk instead of cow's milk), they are following a vegan diet.

Healing

What is healing?

Healing may be spiritual or psychic. Spiritual healing is the healing of the sick in mind, body and spirit. The healing is considered to come from divine energies through prayer and meditation. Psychic healing is similar but has no religious context.

The healer is a person who can harness healing energy, whatever its origin, and can then transfer this energy to the person being healed. It is thought that the transferred energy enhances the recipient's own energy field, or life force, helping to stimulate recovery from the disease or treatment.

What is 'laying on of hands'?

This is a type of spiritual healing involving physical contact between the healer and the person.

Do you have to visit a healer?

No, there are some healers who work at a distance, and so you are not required to visit them.

Is healing available on the NHS?

Healing is not readily available on the NHS. Some healers do not charge a fee but might ask for a donation instead.

Herbalism

What is herbalism?

It is the use of herbs and plants to treat illnesses. Herbal remedies have been used since ancient times to treat a variety of disorders. The whole plant (roots, leaves, stem and seed) is used to make the preparation. Depending on the preparation, it will either be taken orally or be used in ointment form.

Can herbal remedies be used to treat cancer?

They may be used in place of drugs but it is unlikely that cancer can be treated in this way. Some herbs and plants are used in cancer care, such as the painkiller morphia which comes from opium poppies.

Do herbalists have to be trained?

Yes, there is a training course for people who wish to become practitioners.

Homoeopathy

What is homoeopathy?

It is a treatment involving the use of substances known as remedies. These are often made into pills which you dissolve under your tongue. The prescribed remedy aims to help your body to stimulate its own healing process.

The word 'homoeopathy' comes from two Greek words that mean 'similar' and 'suffering'. The remedy that is prepared for you contains a very dilute amount of a substance which in larger quantities would produce similar symptoms to the illness that is being treated. In contrast, most modern medicine works on allopathic principles – 'allopathy' comes from the Greek words for 'other' and 'suffering'. Allopathic treatment has an effect on the body which is opposite to that caused by the disease.

Can homoeopathy be used to treat cancer?

While there is no evidence that homeopathy is helpful for cancer, some people choose to use homoeopathic remedies alone. In practice few doctors recommend homoeopathy as a first treatment choice but might suggest it alongside other treatment.

How does the homoeopath decide on the correct remedy for me?

Your first consultation with a homoeopath will last for at least an hour. During this time you will be asked questions about yourself and your lifestyle, about any physical symptoms you have and any medicine or treatment that has been prescribed for you. You will also be asked about the health of your close relatives both now and in the past. With all this information the homoeopath will then be able to determine which remedy would be the most suitable for you to take.

Is homoeopathy available on the NHS?

Yes it is, but not widely available. Your family doctor should be able to tell you if you can receive homoeopathic treatment on the NHS in the area in which you live.

Do homoeopaths have special training?

All homoeopaths should have gained a recognised qualification in homoeopathy before they practise. Some homoeopaths also have a medical qualification and may have practised as doctors before training to become homoeopaths.

Massage

What is massage?

Massage is a system of treatment for painful muscles, for certain aches, for reducing stiffness, and for helping you to relax. It stimulates the circulation of blood and lymph round the body and this can encourage the removal of waste products and poisons.

Massage can be deep or gentle and the person who gives you the massage may work special oils into your skin which have certain properties that can enhance the effect of the massage. There are many different massage techniques which include kneading, pressing, rubbing, stroking and tapping.

Are there any types of massage which should be avoided by someone who has cancer?

There is some controversy over the suitability of deep massage techniques for people who have cancer. Some people have suggested that the increased blood and lymph circulation that deep massage brings might increase the possibility of cancer being spread from the part of the body being massaged.

Any type of massage which involves vigorous rubbing or kneading or the application of pressure to deeper parts of the body should be avoided, such as Shiatsu massage, which applies pressure to the meridians along which Ch'i flows (see the section on acupuncture for more information about Ch'i).

So which types of massage are suitable for people who have cancer?

Gentle massage, which can be very soothing and relaxing and can help you to feel good, is not likely to affect the cancer.

Aromatherapy and reflexology are probably the two most frequently used professional techniques, but gentle massage could be given to you by a friend at home, if care is taken to avoid the parts of your body where the cancer is or was.

I've heard that massage can be used to treat lymphoedema. What type of massage is this?

Lymphoedema (swelling which can occur due to blockage of the lymph flow following surgery and radiotherapy, for example of the arm after treatment for breast cancer) can be sometimes eased by a combination of techniques which include massage and the use of special compression sleeves. This is not the same as any other types of massage described here. Lymphoedema is discussed more fully in Chapter 5.

Is massage available on the NHS?

Generally speaking, no. Some health professionals may have taken courses in reflexology and may practise it as part of their job. Aromatherapy is, however, gradually becoming more widely available in hospices and some hospitals.

Is there special training for people who want to give massage?

Yes, there are day and evening classes which you can take to learn about aromatherapy or reflexology. There are also longer courses which lead to a formal qualification.

Some people may, however, attend a two day course and then decide to practise massage, so if you are going to seek out aromatherapy or reflexology or any other massage from a professional, be sure to check out their training and qualifications first, to ensure you get someone with suitable experience.

What is aromatherapy?

Aromatherapy is a form of gentle massage treatment using essential oils which come from flowers, roots and leaves. The oils are diluted and massaged into the skin. The aromatherapist will make a mixture of different oils specific for each individual. Often the aromatherapist will play a relaxation tape while giving the massage to help the person to relax.

How can it help people who have cancer?

Combining the effects of gentle massage with the properties of some of the oils can make it an effective tonic for some people.

For example, certain oils can help reduce swelling whereas others may help to strengthen the immune system. It is very important, however, not to have an aromatherapy massage on a part of the body that is receiving or has just had a course of radiotherapy treatment as it might make the skin unnecessarily sore in that area.

Can aromatherapy oils be used in other ways?

Yes, they can. Some oils can be diluted and added to bath water so that you can relax in the bath and gain benefit from the oils. If you have recently had radiotherapy to certain parts of your body, you may have been advised not to have proper baths for a period of time. It is important to observe this and not bathe with oils until you are able to wash as usual.

You can buy burners for essential oils which means that you get the oil vapours released into the room when you use the burner. This can be quite useful for helping you to relax and for trying to combat certain side effects of treatment, such as nausea.

What is reflexology?

It is a type of massage usually given to the feet, although it can be given to the hands. The whole body is seen as being mapped out on the feet – the right side of the body on the right foot and the left side on the left foot. The organs or tissues in a particular body zone are linked to reflex points on the feet (or hands) and massage of these points treats the corresponding part of the body. For example, the liver corresponds to a reflex point towards the outer side of the middle part of the sole of the right foot, and the spleen corresponds to a similar point on the sole of the left foot.

How does it work?

There are different views as to how reflexology works. One view is that the gentle massage helps to improve blood circulation and stimulates the body's immune system. Another is that the body's natural energy flow is blocked by illness or stress and the reflexologist can feel a change in a particular reflex point which corresponds to the blocked part. Massage to this area can remove the blockage so that energy can flow freely again. A possible effect of reflexology is that the massage encourages the body to produce its own painkillers (endorphins) which could lead to fewer painkilling drugs being needed.

If you are going to have an aromatherapy massage, you may find that the aromatherapist starts by giving you a reflexology massage to help to find points of blocked energy to work on and therefore which oils are likely to be most useful.

Can reflexology be useful for people who have cancer?

Yes, it can. Reflexology is not about curing an illness, rather it is focused on eliminating stress and helping people to relax.

Can I practise reflexology at home?

Yes, you can. There are books that you can buy or get from the library that explain the principles of reflexology and how to use it. Perhaps you can learn with a friend so that you can give each other a reflexology massage.

How many sessions are needed for aromatherapy or reflexology to be effective?

That depends on the reason for having it. For some people having just one session can be very beneficial, for others several sessions may be suggested by the therapist to achieve the desired effect.

Meditation

What is meditation?

It is a technique of using your mind in a way that aids relaxation and reduces stress and tension. Some types of meditation have a devotional or religious approach, others such as T'ai Chi have a physical approach. It has been used for centuries and has been a part of both Eastern and Western cultures. In essence, it is based on understanding who we are and how we relate to the universe.

Can it be useful for someone who has cancer?

Yes, meditating regularly can be very useful as it can help to relieve anxiety and the symptoms of stress. It may lead to a person needing to take fewer painkillers, and the combination of all these things can result in an improved quality of life.

How do you learn to meditate?

You could start by reading a book about meditation and trying out some of the basic concentration and breathing techniques. To study further you could go to a teacher experienced in the particular technique you wish to learn. Before learning any meditation technique you will have to learn relaxation techniques.

What happens the first time I go to a teacher?

Well, that varies according to the type of meditation, but you should be told something about meditation and why it might be beneficial. You will then be taught a simple method of meditation.

Is it available on the NHS?

No, but some organisations that teach meditation do not charge.

Do teachers have special training?

The people who teach meditation are not 'trained' but are people who have experience in the technique they practise which they can show you.

Relaxation

What is relaxation?

Relaxation is a technique which can help to improve our quality of life by reducing tension, anxiety and fatigue, and by boosting our bodys' immune systems. Relaxation involves becoming aware of all our muscles and of the tension in them, and then of gradually releasing that tension. Relaxation techniques can be learned either by attending classes or from a pre-recorded cassette.

Can it be useful for people who have cancer?

Yes, it can be useful. For example, some people use relaxation techniques to help them to cope with chemotherapy and radiotherapy.

Is it available on the NHS?

A number of cancer treatment centres have relaxation tapes for you to use. Some may also have a member of staff available to help you to learn the techniques.

Visualisation

What is visualisation?

Once you have learned relaxation techniques, you can learn to see an image in your mind and to alter it as you wish. This is visualisation.

How do I learn how to visualise?

When you learn relaxation techniques you will be taught to picture a scene or an object as part of the relaxation process. Once you are able to create a particular image in this way, you will find you can create new images and make them act in any way you choose.

How can it be helpful for people who have cancer?

Many people find that if they can see their cancer in their mind they can visualise its destruction. For example, some people give their cancer a shape in their mind and imagine it being attacked or engulfed by something. Visualisation can also help some people to cope with the side effects of treatment. They might visualise something cool touching their skin where they have had radiotherapy treatment as a way of helping to soothe skin soreness which can occur as the course of treatment progresses.

Yoga

What is yoga?

It is a combination of relaxation, physical exercises and positions, and breathing control which can lead to physical and psychological well-being.

Is yoga helpful for people who have cancer?

For some people it can be helpful because yoga can improve muscle and joint flexibility. However, it may not be suitable in all types of cancer, and you should check with your doctor and with the yoga teacher before starting to learn. Some teachers ask all pupils to fill in a medical questionnaire before they begin classes. This can enable the teacher to adapt some of the work to make it more suitable for each individual.

Are yoga teachers trained?

Yes, there are training courses for those wishing to teach yoga, although some people will run classes without having received any formal training.

Can I practise yoga on my own once I have been taught?

Certainly you may wish to carry out the exercises at home, but you should be very clear about what you can and can't do because of your cancer. Always check thoroughly with the teacher and possibly with the hospital doctor as well.

Can yoga be adapted to suit me if I can't move quite as before?

Yes, it can. There are books of exercises available that are written specifically for people who have chronic illnesses such as multiple sclerosis or who are in wheelchairs, and an experienced teacher should be able to guide you as well.

If I decide to use a particular complementary therapy, do I still have to go back to the doctor for regular check ups?

Yes! Although you may see a complementary therapist regularly, she or he is not able to carry out medical check ups. Regular check ups are important, as without them your progress cannot be properly monitored. So you should continue going to see whoever is in charge of your aftercare – either the doctor at the hospital follow-up clinic or your family doctor.

5

Immediately after treatment

Introduction

Immediately after treatment for cancer, and in the weeks following the end of a course of therapy, new problems and concerns arise. Some of these are related to the specific treatment which has been received but many are similar for all people with cancer.

Everyone recovers in their own time, and therefore some of the issues discussed here will be early priorities for some people with cancer, while for others they will not become important until much later. Because of this, we have deliberately repeated some information in this chapter and in the following one, which deals with living with cancer in the longer term. If the answers given here are brief, more detailed information will be found in Chapter 6 and vice versa.

Will I have to go back to hospital for check ups?

Yes. The doctor will want to see you at regular intervals to monitor your response to treatment, to observe how it has affected you and to find out how you are adapting to life after your treatment. As time passes these appointments will probably become less frequent, for example changing from once a month to once every three months if all goes well. Each check up will involve several tests to check your general health and to make sure there are no signs of the cancer returning. Waiting for these test results can be an anxious time, even if you are feeling well and have no symptoms. It is natural to worry about what might be found and you might find it helpful to talk to the staff at the hospital about how you are feeling.

Will I feel better immediately after treatment?

You may feel that your health has improved in the weeks following treatment but sometimes it takes longer to recover from the effects of therapy itself. There may be later effects which make you feel you are not getting better as quickly as you would like. There may be times when these delayed effects are similar to the symptoms you experienced before diagnosis and you may fear that your cancer has returned. To avoid this confusion and uncertainty, ask the staff caring for you what you should expect.

Progress is often gradual. You can't recover overnight from a major operation or a course of intensive radiotherapy or chemotherapy. Some days you may think you are back to normal while on others you may feel depressed and tired. This is not unusual.

Now that I'm no longer receiving treatment, will the cancer come back?

It is difficult to say. Obviously everyone hopes that the treatment has either cured the cancer or, if it was known that this was not possible when you started therapy, that it will control the disease for a considerable period of time. In some situations it is easier to predict the outcome than in others.

Will I be able to stop going back for check ups?

This is unlikely. Once you have had cancer the doctors will usually want you to attend for follow-up appointments for the rest of your life. Occasionally they may be confident enough of curing your cancer to discharge you from their care but this depends on the type of cancer you originally had. It is possible that the follow-up checks could be carried out at your local hospital if you had treatment at a specialist hospital or regional centre, or your family doctor may be able to take over your follow-up care.

While I was attending the hospital regularly for treatment, I had hospital transport provided. Can I continue with this?

Possibly. You should talk to your doctor about this. An ambulance or hospital car is only provided if it is necessary on medical grounds. You may find that once treatment is completed and you start to feel better, you can make your own way to and from the hospital by public transport or by driving yourself.

I feel well enough to travel to the hospital but the fares are quite expensive. Can I get any help with them?

Yes, you may be able to get a refund on your fares. You should ask to see a member of the Social Work department who will be able to advise you.

If I continue to need medicines do I have to pay prescription charges each time?

Not necessarily. Discuss this with your doctor or the pharmacy staff. You may be eligible for exemption from prescription charges or you may benefit from buying a season ticket for prescriptions if you are only going to need medicines for a few more months.

What if I need regular supplies of appliances or equipment, do I have to pay for these?

Probably not. Many of the appliances people need are available on prescription and are exempt from charges. You should talk with your doctor, specialist nurse or pharmacist. They will tell you what you need and how to obtain supplies of your particular equipment.

Examples of the items available are colostomy bags, laryngectomy bibs, food supplements, lymphoedema hosiery and incontinence pads. In addition, if you have a breast prosthesis you are entitled to a replacement if it loses its shape or your weight changes. A prosthesis will usually last 2–3 years.

Are there any signs I should look out for which may indicate my cancer has come back?

It is impossible to list the type of things to look for because this depends on your original cancer. Each cancer behaves differently and, if it spreads, may affect different parts of the body. Ask your doctor if there is anything specific of which you should be aware. Generally, you should report any changes in your health or anything which is unusual for you. Not every ache, pain, lump or change will indicate that your cancer has returned, although this may be the first thought that comes to mind. However, report these signs or symptoms to your doctor. If the problem is unrelated to your cancer, your mind will be put at rest and if it is a sign of a recurrence it can be treated as soon as possible.

Is there anything I can do to stop my cancer coming back?

At the moment it is not possible to offer any definite advice but you may feel that you wish to make some changes to your lifestyle to improve your general health and wellbeing.

The doctors say my operation was a success and everyone is pleased with my progress but I can't look at my scar without flinching and I can't accept the changes in my body. Is this normal? How long will it take to adjust?

Your reaction is both normal and natural. Everyone goes through a period of adjustment to change and the time this takes varies from person to person. It often helps to talk about how you are feeling - with your partner, family and friends or one of the staff caring for you. There are many people you can turn to for practical and emotional support. Choose someone with whom you feel comfortable - your hospital doctor, your family doctor, a specialist nurse or someone else you became close to at the hospital. This help and support can be extended to your family if they too are finding it difficult to adjust to what has happened to you. Some hospitals employ trained counsellors with whom you can discuss your feelings and concerns about various aspects of your life.

Remember, even though there may be an outward change in your appearance or body function, you are the same person you were before your treatment for cancer.

I seem to have lost my confidence. When I go out I'm sure everyone knows I've had cancer and I'm different. Is there anything I can do to overcome this?

Many people feel less confident about meeting others, especially if their treatment has resulted in a change in appearance or body function. It takes time to regain your confidence in the same way as it takes time for you to adjust to the changes caused by treatment for cancer. Very often adjustment and self confidence go hand in hand.

If you are in company, the only person who may know of or notice any difference may be you. Friends, colleagues or strangers will only know if you choose to tell them.

You may find it helpful to make contact with a person who has had the same operation or treatment as you. This is possible through many of the support and self help organisations listed in Appendix I.

My operation has affected my speech. Will I be able to use a telephone and will people be able to understand me?

This will depend on the type of operation and how much your speech has been altered. A speech and language therapist will be able to work with you with the aim of regaining as normal a voice as is possible for you. This may take time and patience. It may be necessary for you to use other methods of communication. There are several services and aids provided by BT (British Telecom) which can assist people with communication difficulties.

I've finished my course of chemotherapy but my appetite still hasn't returned. How long will it take before I'm eating normally again?

If your treatment, whatever it was, has affected your appetite it can take a while before you feel that you are enjoying your food as you did previously. This time varies. It is important you eat well to help your recovery but you should not feel that you are forcing yourself to eat. During this time, it may be easier to eat snacks or small meals rather than sitting down to a three course dinner. You can also make use of nourishing drinks. If your loss of appetite persists, ask to see the dietitian who may be able to offer other suggestions.

Can I drink alcohol?

Usually there is no reason why you should not have an occasional drink. A drink before a meal is a good way of perking up your appetite and increasing your calorie (energy) intake. Check with your doctor. It may not be advisable for a time, for example if you have had radiotherapy to your face or neck.

I have a colostomy. I've heard that there are certain foods I should avoid. Is this true?

You should be able to eat a wide variety of foods. Your doctor or stoma care nurse will be able to tell you which foods may affect the function of your colostomy and advise you on how to introduce these gradually into your diet again. You will discover which foods you can or cannot eat by experimenting. There are no hard and fast rules, everyone is different.

After my operation I'm having difficulty chewing and swallowing and I don't think I'm eating enough. What can I do?

The first thing to do is to talk to the staff at the hospital as there are many people who can help you. The dietitian will be able to suggest nourishing foods and drinks which are easier to swallow. The speech and language therapist also helps people who have difficulty swallowing. You may be able to purée or liquidise your favourite foods. If you don't have a liquidiser you may be able to borrow one from the hospital or get some financial help towards buying one.

There are other methods of feeding you if you still have difficulty swallowing. For example, a tube can be passed into your stomach and liquid feeds can be given through this. The tube may only need to be used for a short time and it does not mean you have to stay in hospital, nor will it affect your speech. You can be taught to give your own feeds at home.

During my treatment I lost a lot of weight. Will I get back to normal again?

Your weight loss may have been due to your cancer as well as the treatment you have had. Now your cancer has been treated you should be able to regain your weight but this may take time. Ask to see a dietitian who will be able to advise you what to eat so that you take in enough protein and energy-containing foods to increase your weight.

I had a laryngectomy and now I suffer from constipation, which I never did before. Why is this?

When we open our bowels, we strain by closing our larynx and holding our breath. Because you can no longer do this you are more likely to become constipated. You can avoid the problem by eating more high-fibre foods such as cereals containing bran, wholemeal bread, baked beans and fruit. If you continue to have a problem with this contact the dietitian for advice or speak to your doctor who can prescribe a laxative.

Towards the end of my radiotherapy I suffered from diarrhoea, which is still a problem. What should I do?

Your bowel has been irritated by the radiation and will gradually recover. Continue to follow the advice you were given during treatment, avoiding foods which contain a lot of roughage and drinking plenty of fluids. If diarrhoea continues to be troublesome ask your doctor or dietitian for further suggestions or medication.

Should I try to avoid putting on weight?

In general, yes. If you have had a breast implant or have had a stoma formed, it is better not to put on too much weight because it may change your appearance or affect the ease with which you can change your appliance. However, if you have lost weight you will obviously want to get back to your normal weight after your treatment.

I've been on steroids as part of my therapy. How soon can I expect to lose the weight I've gained?

The speed at which you lose weight will depend on how long you have been taking steroids and the dose you have been taking. You will probably notice some weight loss within the first couple of weeks as the fluid which has been retained leaves your body. The remaining extra weight will be lost more gradually.

I used to exercise to keep fit and control my weight. How long will it be before I can start again?

It is difficult to give a definite time, for example four weeks or two months – it will depend on how you feel. When you begin to exercise again, increase your activities gradually and don't push yourself too hard. You might like to start with a daily walk, increasing the distance as you feel more fit. Gentle swimming can be relaxing and provides good, all-round exercise.

Can anyone go swimming?

The general answer to this is yes but some people need to take special precautions or will have special concerns.

If you have had a laryngectomy, you will need training and special equipment to prevent water entering your stoma. You should contact the **National Association of Laryngectomee Clubs** for information about courses in swimming; the address is in Appendix I.

If you have received radiotherapy, you should check with your doctor. Your skin will remain sensitive for a time after treatment and may be irritated by chlorine in swimming pools.

If you have had a mastectomy, you may feel less confident about going swimming. Your breast care nurse or the **Breast Care and Mastectomy Association** can offer advice on how to adapt swimming costumes and where to buy special swimwear; the address is in Appendix I.

If you have a colostomy or other stoma you may also feel apprehensive about swimming. However, there is no reason to be. Your stoma care nurse or the **British Colostomy Association** can offer practical advice about suitable appliances to wear; the address is in Appendix I.

If you, or your child, have a Hickman catheter still in place following chemotherapy treatment you should check with the doctor before going swimming.

Ask for advice if you are unsure about whether you should swim or not.

After my operation I was given special exercises to do by the physiotherapist. How long do I need to continue these?

You should ask your physiotherapist when you may stop any special exercises. The physiotherapist will have planned these individually for you to prevent stiffness, to increase your range of movement or to improve your muscle strength. Don't stop the exercises without checking first, or you may not gain the full benefit from them and problems may occur later.

I haven't been able to do very much around the house. When can I begin doing shopping and housework?

Generally, when you feel able to. Housework is a more energetic activity than we tend to think so start slowly with dusting, washing-up and cooking light meals. Gradually add in other activities such as vacuuming, ironing and going out shopping. If you have had an operation (for example, a hysterectomy, bowel surgery or a mastectomy) you will usually be given specific advice by the doctor or physiotherapist about what you can and cannot do in the weeks after surgery. In most cases energetic activities should be avoided for at least six weeks but do not worry if it takes longer before you feel back to normal. Everyone recovers at their own pace.

Does gardening provide you with good exercise?

Yes, and it gets you out into the fresh air. However, you should start with light jobs like weeding and not try to dig the vegetable patch or mow the lawn in one go. If you have had a mastectomy you will be advised to wear gloves while gardening. This is because a proportion of women may develop lymphoedema (swelling) of the arm on the side that has received treatment. A scratch could lead to an infection and this could trigger off the swelling.

What is lymphoedema?

Lymphoedema is the collection of fluid in the tissues under the skin. This fluid causes swelling and may affect a limb or a part of the body. Lymph is a colourless liquid which is formed by the tissues of the body. It is normally taken back into the bloodstream through the small tubes and glands which make up the lymphatic system. These tubes and glands may be damaged by treatment for cancer and so the lymph cannot drain away. This results in oedema (swelling).

Can lymphoedema be prevented?

It is not usually possible to prevent lymphoedema. However, your doctor can tell you if there is a chance that you may develop it after your surgery or radiotherapy for cancer. The doctor, physiotherapist and nursing staff will also be able to suggest ways in which you can reduce the likelihood of developing lymphoedema.

Can lymphoedema be treated?

Yes. Much more is now known about why lymphoedema develops and how it can be treated. Several methods are used to control swelling including special massage techniques and elastic support sleeves or stockings. Treatment will be more effective if it is started as soon as any swelling is noticed. Even if swelling is mild or comes and goes, report it to your doctor.

More information about lymphoedema can be found in a booklet called **Lymphoedema – Advice on Treatment**. Details are given in Appendix II.

My husband and I are about to move house. Will I be able to help with this?

There is no reason why you should not be able to help. The golden rule is not to do too much and leave the heavy work to someone else. After treatment for cancer, especially if this has included an operation, you will often be advised not to lift heavy items, carry heavy shopping or pick up young children, who can be surprisingly heavy, for a couple of months afterwards. If someone has had a laryngectomy, it may not be possible to lift heavy objects because in order to do this we normally hold our breath and the means to do this no longer exists.

Sometimes I sit down to read a book or write a letter and find I can't concentrate. Is this normal?

Lack of concentration is not uncommon. It may be due to the

effects of treatment or simply because you have not fully adjusted to having a serious illness. Usually when we are ill, even if it's just a bout of flu, we feel mentally less alert and less able to concentrate. If you don't feel you are recovering as quickly as you should, it may help to talk to someone about this. It may set your mind at rest that you are not unusual.

How soon after treatment can I start driving again?

You should discuss this with your doctor. Illness and treatment may affect your concentration and reflexes. In addition your physical movements may be restricted or a seat belt may cause discomfort to a part of your body, such as your chest or abdomen. You may be able to drive within weeks or months of finishing your therapy but in some circumstances, for example treatment for a brain tumour, it may be much longer. If you drive when your doctor has advised you not to, your insurance will be invalidated.

What is 'somnolence syndrome'?

Somnolence syndrome is the name given to a group of symptoms which are later effects of radiotherapy. It usually occurs between six and 10 weeks after the end of treatment. Adults or children who have received radiotherapy to the brain or who have had total body irradiation (TBI) before a bone marrow transplant may experience these effects. For a period of about a week you will feel lethargic, tired, sleepy and, occasionally, depressed. Everything is too much of an effort, even small things you have been able to do until that time. There is no way this syndrome can be prevented or treated. It is not a permanent setback and does not mean your cancer has come back. However, it can be frightening if you do not expect it to occur. Your doctor, radiographers or nurses will tell you if you are likely to experience somnolence.

When can I start picking up the threads of my social life again?

Whenever you feel ready to do so. The time you choose will depend on how you feel physically, how confident you are about mixing with other people and what you want to do. The important thing is not to overtire yourself by doing too much too soon.

Is there anything I shouldn't do?

Not really, but check with your doctor if you are in any doubt.

Occasionally, a person will be given specific advice which may only need to be followed for a short time or which may be relevant in the long term. For example, if you have had chemotherapy, or any other treatment which has affected your blood count, you may be advised to avoid crowded places for a while because you are still at risk of picking up an infection more easily. If you have had an operation on your chest or a laryngectomy you may be advised to avoid smoky or dusty surroundings which can cause irritation and affect your breathing. Any operation on your stomach or bowel may limit how much and what type of food you wish to eat when you go out for a meal.

These recommendations will be particular to your cancer, its treatment and effects, and to you as an individual. Ask your doctor if you are unsure about what you can do or how soon you can take up social activities again.

I don't have the energy to go out with friends or do the things I did before treatment. I don't feel I'm achieving anything, what can I do?

Any illness unsettles your normal routine and if you are used to being busy it is very frustrating when you don't feel able to take part in your usual activities. Recovery, both physical and emotional, is gradual. You may have up days and down days. Try to take advantage of the days when you have more energy and plan activities in advance so that you can use these times effectively. Even if you don't feel like going out, family and friends can visit or you might like to take up a new hobby, something you always wanted to do but never had time for.

When can I return to work?

This will depend to a large extent on what your job entails. You may have continued working, full-time or part-time, during your treatment. If you were unable to work, discuss the possibility of returning on a part-time basis with your employer. If you have been working part-time during treatment you may be able to go back full-time quite soon.

If your job is mentally stressful or involves heavy manual work you may need a longer interval between finishing therapy and resuming your employment.

Depending on how you feel, you might wish to discuss this with your doctor, your occupational health department at work or your employer to help you come to a decision.

When can my child go back to school?

It's difficult to say. Your child may recover quickly and be impatient to return to school and the company of friends. You should discuss this with the doctor because even if treatment is finished and no obvious side effects are present, there may be other reasons why a delay is desirable. However, this delay does not mean school work has to suffer. Your child may be able to study at home and enjoy contact with friends, providing they are free from colds or other infections.

Is there any reason why I can't go on holiday?

No, it's a good idea to plan a holiday or short break as soon as you feel well enough but you may have to take some extra factors into consideration, for example checking whether you have sufficient supplies of medicines or appliances for the time you are away. If you wish to travel abroad, ask your doctor if there are any countries it is unwise to visit, perhaps because of the risk of an infection. In many countries medical supervision can be arranged and your doctor can provide a letter containing details of your illness, in case you need care while on holiday.

Is it all right to go sunbathing?

As a general rule whenever you sunbathe you should protect your skin with a sunblock cream and avoid the hottest time of the day. If you have received radiotherapy to any part of your body, that area should be protected as the skin will be more sensitive. Some chemotherapy agents (for example 5FU, Methotrexate and Actinomycin) can also increase the sensitivity of your skin and may cause an unusual darkening of the skin. If you have received these drugs you should be particularly sure to avoid bright sunlight. Check with your doctor and observe all the usual recommendations to protect your skin from the sun.

How soon can I resume sexual activity?

This varies from individual to individual. The doctors will offer definite guidance in some situations, for example after a hysterectomy or removal of a bladder tumour by cystoscopy, but very often it is left up to you to decide when, and if, you wish to resume sexual activity.

If you have simply lost interest in sex during your illness and treatment, you will probably find your feelings return once you are well again and have adapted to the physical and emotional changes caused by your treatment. You may find sexual activity more tiring or difficult at first, but this will improve with time.

A change in body appearance may cause concerns about loss of attractiveness, femininity or masculinity. Talking to your partner about these feelings may help to dispel them. You may wish to discuss your thoughts and fears with others, such as a specialist nurse or a counsellor. Do not be embarrassed about this, it is an important aspect of your recovery and adjustment.

Practical problems may result from your treatment, such as vaginal dryness or scarring after radiotherapy in women or difficulty in maintaining an erection in men. You will be given advice on how to prevent or reduce these problems, for example on how to use a vaginal dilator to prevent the vaginal walls sticking together immediately following radiotherapy. Because of these practical difficulties your partner may be scared of hurting you or failing to satisfy you. Patience may be required and your relationship may resume more slowly. There are many ways of meaningful love making and pleasurable sexual contact. You may find that this is the time to explore them.

It may be that your surgery or other therapy has permanently affected your sexual function. You may need specialist advice or counselling regarding these changes and how to cope with them.

Now all my treatment is finished and I'm not going back to the hospital so often, I feel really alone. Who can I talk to?

Firstly, even though you are no longer attending hospital, it doesn't mean you can't get in touch with the staff there. If you have concerns of a medical nature, you should contact your doctor straight away so that you do not worry unnecessarily.

Secondly, many hospitals now have specialist nurses or other staff with whom you can discuss practical and emotional problems. Frequently these staff will encourage you to telephone if you are feeling low or have questions about what is happening. If you wish to take advantage of their offer, then do so – they really do mean what they say.

Thirdly, you may find you are more comfortable talking with your family doctor whom you may have known for a long time and who also knows your family well. Some practices also have specialist community nurses or counsellors attached to them, who may be able to help and support you.

How can I find someone who really understands how I feel?

There are numerous voluntary organisations which have been set up by people with cancer and their families, or by other individuals who have a common interest in a particular aspect of health or illness. Details of these organisations are given in Appendix I. Some of them offer a confidential telephone service, providing information and support. Others can give you a list of local support and self-help groups, if you wish to meet with people in your own area, or they may have a network of people throughout the country who you can talk with or meet on an individual basis. There are many people who have been through a similar experience of cancer and treatment, who will understand how you feel. Parents of children with cancer and other members of a family can also find contacts and support in this way.

What's the difference between a support group and a self help group?

It's probably easier to think first of the similarities rather than the differences. In fact the two terms are often interchangeable. Both are places where people can go to meet others who are going through or have been through similar experiences. Self help groups, however, are generally only for the person who has had cancer, whereas support groups may be open to anyone affected by cancer in any way, that is friends and relatives too.

I don't want to sit around listening to everyone describing what happened to them. Isn't this what happens in a support group?

No. People go to groups for lots of different reasons. Often the most important one is to meet people who have been through a similar experience to themselves. Being amongst people who can really identify with you and your experience can be very strengthening and positive. In such company many people feel they can relax and that they don't have to be concerned about putting on a brave face for their friends or family.

Support groups usually offer a variety of activities which may include:

(i)   regular meetings with an invited speaker followed by time to chat;
(ii)   regular 'drop-in' times for people to get together with no formal structure;
(iii) the opportunity to try certain complementary therapies;
(iv)   counselling or befriending;
(v)   social events.

There are also support networks in which a person who is in a particular situation can receive telephone or written support from someone else who is in the same situation and they may never meet face to face.

For many people, being part of a support group or network helps them to live with cancer. For information about organisations that can help you find support turn to Appendix I.

6
Life with and after cancer

Introduction

Having cancer is going to affect your lifestyle, both during and after treatment. You will probably feel a wide range of emotions as the impact of being told you have cancer hits you. The reactions of people close to you, such as friends or relatives, will also affect you.

There may be things which you decide to alter in your life as a result of having cancer. There may be things which you have to alter, and for which you need to make some adjustments.

Until quite recently, little attention was given to helping people cope with having cancer. Now, practical, emotional and psychological support are all available for someone who has cancer, as well as for friends and relatives.

Why me?

Probably everyone who develops cancer asks this question. Many people ask it when they first hear that they have cancer (or suspect they have it), and may ask it repeatedly during any treatment and beyond. One of the hardest things for anyone else to do is to provide an answer, because there isn't one, single explanation. Why you should have cancer at this point in your life is unlikely to be known. The many theories as to what causes different types of cancer are discussed in Chapter 1. This does not necessarily provide any comfort at a time when you are likely to be feeling many mixed emotions. And the last thing you

114

are likely to find helpful is to be told 'not to worry' or to 'put on a brave face' or to feel you have to keep your own feelings inside you to 'protect' others.

Why has this happened to my child?

Once again this is a very common and important question which does not have a clear answer. Whatever the age of your child, as a parent you are likely to have many questions and to feel very angry, sad, shocked, guilty and unable to believe it to be true. Many parents talk of wishing it was happening to them instead. People often find it particularly hard to accept that a young child or teenager has cancer and might have to face gruelling treatment. Yet often the child or teenager comes to accept their illness and may cope better than the parents. It may be important for you to acknowledge that your child could help you to accept what has happened, and that you can provide each other with mutual support.

Should I make any changes to my lifestyle after having cancer?

Many people ask whether they should do anything different after they have had cancer. Certainly there are things you can do that can reduce your chances of getting another cancer in the future. Having come through the emotional minefield that cancer often brings with it, and having got through treatment and any side effects, many people view their future in a different light.

A sense of being a survivor and perhaps of being given a second chance can lead to you wanting to do things that may not have occurred to you before.

Talking about cancer

How can I find someone to talk to who has been through something similar?

There are several ways in which you can find support or share your experiences, feelings, hopes and fears with people who may have been in a similar situation.

(i)   By making contact with a local cancer support and self help group (see Appendix I for information about how to find a local group). Groups may be specifically for people who have a particular type of cancer, or they may be open to anyone who has any type of cancer. Some groups are only for the person who has the cancer but many include relatives and friends too, and there are special support groups for parents of young children and teenagers. Group activities vary from regular meetings, perhaps with a speaker, to social events. How often a group meets and the time of day varies from group to group.

(ii) By speaking to someone on the telephone. There are organisations that provide information over the phone about cancer and its treatment. They have trained staff who can give you the time and space to talk, as well as trying to help you to find answers to any questions. They can also help you to work out the questions you would like to ask your doctor, for example. If you choose to telephone such an organisation you can remain anonymous and talk in confidence. Some organisations are willing to call you back to save you the cost of a long phone call; others operate a freephone system.

(iii) By asking at the hospital where you go for treatment. Some hospitals know of local people who have been treated there or who attend clinics for check ups, and who are willing to come in and talk with you.

I've got cancer. Should I talk about what is happening or not?

That is for you to decide. Some people choose right at the start to talk openly and honestly to their partner or relatives or close friends or work colleagues. Through this they are able to share the feelings they experience and can gain support and strength to cope with what is happening. Other people prefer not to talk about what is going on. They may cope well with what is happening but sometimes it can be hard for others to deal with their silence about the subject. Partners, relatives and friends will have their own feelings about what is happening to you and how it affects them, and problems can arise if your cancer becomes a taboo subject that must not be mentioned.

I want to talk about things but it's hard to know where to start. What if I cry?

Many people think that if they allow themselves to cry in front of someone else they will cause greater distress to themselves and to the other person. While it can be very painful to let yourself cry 'in public' it can be very beneficial in the end. Bottling up feelings means they will probably force their way out sooner or later and in a way that might be less within your control. Having cancer is an extremely emotional experience but sharing those feelings, rather than keeping them all inside, can relieve some of the tension and enable you to face whatever lies ahead in the most constructive way possible, with support and understanding from people who are important to you.

It is at this time that many people contact a cancer support and information organisation. Talking in private on the phone to a person you don't know and aren't likely to meet can give you the chance to have a practice run through of things that you might want to say to a friend or relative. This can make it easier for you when you do talk with them.

What should I tell my children?

Children are likely to notice if you are not quite your usual self, and may feel they are in some way to blame if they are not given some sort of explanation. Exactly what you tell them will probably depend first and foremost on their ages, but as a general rule it is likely to be better for the whole household in the long run if you can tell them as much of the truth as possible. You may wish to tell it to them gradually over a period of time or you may tell an older child more in the first instance than a younger child, although the older child may then tell the younger one anyway! If you are going to be having treatment that could make you quite ill, or if you are going to be in hospital, you may also find it helpful to tell your children's teachers, so that they are aware and can help to support the child in their class.

My son has cancer. What should I tell my other children?

Once again being as honest and open as possible is likely to be the best approach, taking age into account. The other children might feel jealous that their brother is getting lots of extra attention if they do not understand why. Or they might be anxious that the same thing could happen to them. After all, they all caught chickenpox off each other ... so they may need a lot of reassurance. Your children's teachers should also be kept in the picture for the reasons mentioned in the previous question.

You might find you have to spend a great deal of time at the hospital with your son, and so may need to ask people to pick up the other children from school or to be at your home with them. If you do not have anyone you can ask to help in this way, you may find it useful to contact a local cancer support group to see if they can help. You could also ask to see a social worker at the hospital to explain your situation and see if they can suggest any other avenues to explore. Don't be afraid to ask.

Diet

Is it true that eating some foods increases the risk of cancer?

There have been many research projects which have looked at the links between certain cancers and foods. To give just a couple of examples, it appears that breast cancer is more likely to occur in populations that traditionally have a diet with a high fat content, whereas cancer of the nasopharynx (the area behind the nose and mouth) seems to be more common in populations that eat large quantities of smoked foods. The studies are helpful generalisations, but just because they high-light certain links, it does not mean that you, as an individual, are necessarily going to develop a particular cancer because of your diet.

Why do I have to eat a well balanced diet after I have had cancer?

A balanced diet is better for your general health. For most of us, eating a better balanced diet means having less fatty food, cutting down on our salt intake and eating more fibre (roughage) in the form of fresh vegetables and cereals. Eating this type of diet is good for everyone, not just for people who have had cancer. For example, eating plenty of high-fibre foods can help to prevent constipation and other bowel disorders and may also reduce the chances of getting bowel cancer.

A balanced diet will make sure that you get the vitamins and minerals you need to help your body to recover from any treatment you have had and to build you up again. If you can't face full meals have several snacks instead, and eat as and when you fancy something rather than at set meal times.

What if I just can't eat?

Some people find that because of the side effects they experience from their treatment they are unable to eat as they usually would and have to adapt their diet for some weeks. Some people may have to adapt their diet permanently as a result of their cancer or treatment. In both of these cases, a hospital dietitian would be a good person to consult, because they will be able to identify foods which you could eat to get the nutrients you need. Some of the organisations listed in Appendix I may also be able to provide you with some ideas about what you could eat.

What about complementary diets?

People may choose to follow a particular complementary diet when they have cancer and to continue with this when hospital treatment is finished. If you wish to try a new eating plan which is very different from your usual diet, make sure you let the hospital doctor know what you are planning. This is because some diets could prolong and increase the severity of certain side effects of treatment, such as diarrhoea, and so it might be better to wait until these are over before changing to a new style of eating. Information about some specific complementary diets can be found in Chapter 4.

Will changing my diet help to prevent my cancer from getting worse?

There is no scientific evidence to suggest that changing your diet would do this.

Will changing my diet reduce the chances of my cancer coming back?

Again there is no scientific evidence to suggest this. However, by changing to a more healthy, balanced diet you will be helping to improve your body's general condition and your general health, which may have an impact on the cancer.

Drinking alcohol

What about drinking alcohol after having a course of treatment for cancer?

Depending on the cancer and treatment you have had, you might be finding it hard to swallow. Alcohol can aggravate this, so it is better not to drink at all until the side effects have passed. You should also avoid excessive alcohol completely as it is not good for your general health, but an occasional glass of something is unlikely to be harmful.

Could drinking alcohol have caused my cancer?

There are thought to be links between drinking – spirits in particular – and some cancers of the mouth, throat and liver, to name a few examples. It is also possible that women who regularly drink 2–3 units of alcohol a day have an increased risk of developing breast cancer compared with women who do not drink. (One unit of alcohol is equal to one glass of wine or one pub measure of spirits or half a pint of beer, cider or lager.)

Research into these links is continuing. There is no evidence yet to show that drinking alcohol increases the risk of cancer coming back.

Smoking

I've got cancer. Should I stop smoking?

Whilst the strict medical answer to this is often going to be 'yes', it is not quite that simple. If you have cancer, then you may want to adopt a new approach to life in general which could include giving up smoking. On the other hand, you may feel that that there is little point in stopping smoking once you have cancer and that attempting to do so could add to the stress caused by the illness.

Having had cancer, should I stop smoking?

That is really something for you to decide. There are known links between certain cancers, such as lung cancer, and smoking, but it is also true that people who have never smoked can get lung cancer. If giving up smoking is going to affect you adversely, then you may prefer not to stop. If you do continue to smoke you could try to cut down and change to a very low tar brand of cigarette or cigar.

Exercise

What about taking exercise during treatment and after it has finished?

Exercise is good to stimulate the heart and to tone up flabby muscle, but you should be careful not to start to do too much too soon during treatment or after it has finished, as you do not want to make yourself overtired. Gentle, regular exercise throughout your treatment and beyond is far better for your body than sudden, strenuous activity when treatment is over.

Are there any forms of exercise which are better than others following treatment?

It is well known that swimming is a good way of exercising your whole body. However, you should avoid swimming if, for example, you have recently completed a course of radiotherapy

– your skin will be sensitive on the part of your body that was treated, and chlorine from a pool could make any skin reaction to treatment worse.

In general, if you are used to doing one particular type of exercise, then you may wish to continue with it. You might need to modify how much you do to take account of the fact that your body is not quite back to its usual state. Check with your doctor if you have any questions about what your limits should be.

Weight

I've got cancer. Is it important to watch my weight?

Yes, it is. Having cancer might mean that you gain weight or you might lose weight.

There are links between being overweight and an increased risk of getting breast cancer, and there are also links between obesity and both cancer of the endometrium (lining of the womb) and cancer of the gallbladder. Even if the type of cancer you have is not one of these, you might want to try to watch your weight as this can help to reduce the chances of getting another cancer in the future.

If you have lost weight through having cancer, you might want to try to build yourself up again so that you can get back to your usual self. Excessive weight loss is likely to leave you feeling weak. This could leave you open to infections and other illnesses, and it could take you a longer time to get over the effects of any treatment you have had.

The Sun

Can I sit out in the sun after I've had cancer?

That depends on the cancer and the treatment. Radiotherapy treatment will lead to the skin in the area that was treated being more sensitive than before. As long as this part of the body is kept covered and has sunblock cream on it as well, then it is not likely to burn if you go out in the sun. This applies for at least a couple of years after treatment, and perhaps for longer if you have fair skin.

In any case it is not advisable for anyone to sit out in the sun for very long periods of time. Try to avoid the hottest part of the day as well, when the sun is at its most fierce.

Can I swim in the sea or a pool if it is sunny?

If you are swimming when there is strong sunlight, you should put on a waterproof sunblock and then cover up any treated area if possible. For example, you could wear a T-shirt if the treated area was on your chest. Better still, avoid the strongest sunlight. Remember to take care even if it is cloudy, as the sun's rays still filter through.

I know there are links between skin cancer and sunlight, but are the risks increased if I've had cancer?

The links between prolonged exposure to the sun and skin cancers (although they often do not develop for many years to come) are still present but are not increased if you have had cancer.

Holidays

Can I go on holiday straight after having treatment?

There isn't a simple answer to this. It depends on the cancer and the treatment you have had and you might want to ask your doctor's opinion before making a decision.

It can be very beneficial to get away and rest in order to build yourself up again. However, you may find you are still likely to experience some side effects and so you may want to wait a little longer before taking a break. This will depend on when you finished your treatment and what the treatment was.

If you are planning to go to a hot climate do take notice of the points mentioned in the previous questions about the sun.

Is it safe for me to have a vaccination before I go on holiday?

If you have recently had treatment, particularly chemotherapy, your body's defence (immune) system is quite likely to be weakened. Some vaccinations (for example, those to protect against smallpox or cholera, which are known as active vaccinations) involve the introduction of a small amount of the virus into your body. This stimulates your body's own defence system to develop protection against the disease. If your defence system is not fully recovered from the effects of the treatment then it is not going to be able to react to the vaccination in the normal way, and it is likely that you will be ill. Before you plan to go to any country that would require you to have any sort of vaccination or medication, you should check with the doctor who has treated your cancer to see if it is safe to proceed. This might still apply a few months after treatment has finished.

If I need regular medication, can I take it abroad with me?

Yes, generally speaking you can, providing that you take with you a letter of explanation from your doctor. The letter should be written on headed notepaper from the hospital or practice. Make sure that you have more than enough medication in case of unforseen delays.

Before booking a holiday, you should check with the doctor, and perhaps with the country's embassy, just in case the country you are going to would impose restrictions because of the type of medication you are having. For example, if you are taking strong painkillers, some countries might confiscate these when you arrive, if you have not got the correct paperwork. The correct paperwork, however, may not guarantee that they still would not be taken away from you.

Can I get insurance for my holiday?

Yes, there is special holiday and travel insurance available for people who have had cancer. If you are booking a holiday through a travel agent be sure to check the small print in any insurance cover offered to you because you may find you are excluded from some of the cover. Some of the organisations listed in Appendix I will be able to provide you with more information about holiday insurance.

What happens if I'm taken ill while I'm away?

It is difficult to give a precise answer. It will largely depend on what the illness is and where you are. As a general guide any condition that requires hospitalisation or prolonged treatment would probably best be treated in this country if you can travel home. If you have any doubts about any treatment offered to you while away, insist that contact is made with your doctor. If you do come back because of an illness, ensure that your family doctor and hospital doctor are informed. This is because even if the illness is not related to the cancer, there may be some treatments that are more suitable than others.

If I need to have treatment abroad, do I have to pay for it?

Yes, but there are a number of countries that have a reciprocal agreement with the UK which means that you can have treatment in that country, pay and be reimbursed by the Department of Health when you return.

Sex and relationships

Does having cancer mean I have to stop having a sex life?

No, it does not. While many people find that they are quite tired during and immediately after a course of treatment, once the side effects have passed their desire for a sexual relationship and their interest in sex returns. If you feel you want to have sex then why not? You should be quite gentle, however, if the treatment you have had was to any of the sexual organs. The emotional impact of cancer can play a large part in when and whether or not you want to have sex, and this is discussed later in this chapter.

Can treatment affect my ability to have sex?

Yes, it can. Different treatments can affect this in different ways, some being more obvious than others. Radiotherapy and surgery in the pelvic region can sometimes cause temporary or permanent damage to nerves and tissues in that area. An operation to remove your voice box (laryngectomy) will mean you cannot breathe in the same way as before. This will affect your ability to have an orgasm.

Is there anything I can do to improve the situation?

If there are physical reasons as to why you might have problems with having sex, there are some practical solutions you can try – see the answers to the next three questions. Accepting that there may be problems and discussing these with your partner can help to reduce any anxieties that you may have and can take off some of the pressure when you do try to have sex again. Whatever you do, if you have both had the chance to talk about your respective anxieties, you may find ways of lessening them. For example, you might agree to concentrate on touching and stroking each other.

I've been told that treatment might scar my vagina. What will this do to me? What can I do about it?

A woman may find that her vagina and cervix are scarred after radiotherapy or surgery to the pelvic region. This can mean that the tissues are not as elastic as before, making it difficult and painful to have a penis or fingers inserted into the vagina. Her natural vaginal secretions may dry up, at least temporarily, which will cause further discomfort.

In some cases, the problems will be temporary and will gradually disappear. It is possible to use vaginal dilators to gradually stretch your vagina again. You should start with a small size dilator and gradually work up to larger sizes. Alternatively, you (or your partner) could use your fingers to stretch your vagina. Start by gently inserting one finger and when this becomes easier to do over a period of time, try inserting two fingers and, later on, three fingers.

If your vaginal secretions have dried up, you may find it helpful to use a lubricant like KY Jelly to make having sex more comfortable. You should use a lubricant if you are using a vaginal dilator and it may also be helpful if you are using fingers to stretch your vagina.

Some operations will involve the total removal of a woman's vagina. In these cases an artificial vagina can be constructed by a specialist surgeon.

I've been told I might be impotent after treatment. Is there anything I can do about this?

Impotence means that a man has difficulty in having and maintaining an erection. In many cases the impotence is only temporary, but it can take a couple of years before you are back to how you were before your operation. It is quite likely that you will find your erection is weaker than before but this often improves with time. If impotence does become a long-term problem, there are now various forms of treatment available, including vacuum devices (which look like rigid condoms) and injections of papaverine into the penis. It is also possible to have a penile prosthesis (implant). You can find out about these from your doctor who may refer you to another specialist.

There may be additional problems for men who have anal intercourse. The anus may have been closed by surgery, or it may have been part of an area treated by radiotherapy, in which case it will probably become sore and lose some of its elasticity, at least temporarily. It may be possible to gently dilate the anus using fingers and a lubricant as the side effects begin to pass.

Will I be able to have an orgasm after my laryngectomy?

It is likely that once you have learned how to adapt the way you breathe, you will find you can experience orgasms again, although they may not be quite the same as before.

Do some people stop wanting to have sex completely?

Yes, they do. It is quite usual for people to lose their interest in sex temporarily, during and after treatment. Often, though, their libido returns gradually.

Can my partner catch cancer off me through sex?

No, your partner can not catch cancer from you. Cancer is not a disease that is transmitted by sexual contact or by contact between body fluids.

How can I ever get used to what has happened to my body?

Many people say this. If the cancer or treatment have caused physical changes to your body, you will need time to adjust to these, both physically and emotionally. Some people find that talking to their partner about how they are feeling can help. Others might prefer to see a specialist counsellor, go along to a cancer support group or talk to a specialist health professional such as a stoma care nurse.

If you are able to share your feelings you may find it can help you to start to come to terms with what has happened, which in turn can be a big part of the recovery process.

The changes brought about by the cancer and/or treatment can lead to people not wanting to undress in front of anyone else, let alone have sex with another person. This is very common and for many people adapting to the changes that have happened can take time. It is another of the reasons why many people find that talking things through can help.

Who should I talk to?

Whoever you feel most comfortable with. You may want to talk to a friend rather than your partner, or to a professional counsellor. If you have contact with a local cancer support group you might feel that is the place to go to talk through your feelings. You may choose to phone a cancer helpline where you can remain anonymous.

It's all too personal and I don't want to talk to anyone. Does this mean I'm not helping myself?

No. Many people feel uncomfortable about talking to anyone about things related to sex or relationships or about emotional matters, whether or not they have had cancer. If you find that there are thoughts that keep going round and round in your head, then you might find it helpful to write them all down – your fears and your worries and your hopes. By transferring what is in your head onto paper, even if you tear it up and throw it away immediately afterwards, you may find it helps you to get matters clear and to free your mind to think about other things.

I've had cancer and treatment that has affected my face. How can I ever cope with this?

The effects of such treatment can be devastating and it can be extremely hard to imagine going out and coping with being looked at, even if you have a good prosthesis. It can be very hard, too, for people close to you to cope with such visible changes and this is bound to have an impact on the relationship you have with your partner. People do cope with these changes, with help and support and time. There is a special support network for the facially disfigured called **Let's Face It** listed in Appendix I.

I've had a laryngectomy. Will I learn to speak properly again?

Yes, there are different ways of speaking and people who have a total laryngectomy are often taught to speak by a speech and language therapist. There are permanent prostheses in the form of valves that can be implanted into the neck which can aid speech. It is usually possible with training and perseverance to develop a good enough oesophageal voice technique to enable you to talk on the telephone. There are also 'artificial larynxes' which are vibrating devices held against the neck but these do not produce as good quality speech.

How can I learn to live with a colostomy?

Everyone who has an operation that will result in a colostomy will be shown how to manage the practicalities of changing the bag before they leave hospital. In most cases a specialist stoma care nurse will be the person who will help you to do this. There are different types of appliances and you may need to try a few to find the one that suits you best.

Coming to terms with the emotional impact of having a colostomy can take some time. Many people talk of being afraid to go out of their homes in case the bag leaks, or of feeling embarrassed to go swimming, or of being very self-conscious about the bag showing under their clothes. It may seem hard to believe at first, but most people will never notice your bag.

Some people find that others try to protect them and won't let children or pets jump onto their lap. Usually, given time, friends and relatives will adjust to your stoma and learn to live with it, just as you will. There are specialist organisations that can help you talk through any problems or anxieties that you may have and these are listed in Appendix I.

Will I ever be able to get used to having to use a breast prosthesis?

At first, coping with the emotional effect of losing your breast through cancer can feel like a huge hurdle to get over. Using a prosthesis in your bra to provide you with the external appearance of having two breasts can be useful in helping you to face the outside world.

The permanent breast prostheses come in different shapes and sizes but unfortunately the range of colour available is limited. One manufacturer of breast prostheses will, however, tint any style in their range to a colour that is close to the woman's natural skin and another manufacturer has produced a range of off-the-shelf prostheses for black women. It is also possible for women who have had a partial mastectomy to get a shell in either pink or brown. Being able to select a prosthesis that resembles your own skin colour tones can be a good boost to your self-esteem.

Wearing a properly fitted prosthesis can also give you the confidence to wear evening dresses, tops with thin straps and swimwear. It is possible to buy special swimwear, for example, into which you can insert your prosthesis, knowing it will not slip out of place. The first time you try to wear something like this, you may be quite self-conscious, but it usually gets easier after the first time.

It may take you a long time to feel that you can look at your chest and see the effects of the operation you have had. This is quite common, and is one of the reasons why talking about your feelings and fears to someone else who has been through a similar operation can be helpful. There are many cancer support groups specifically for women who have had breast cancer as well as specialist organisations that can provide you with emotional support and practical information. Their addresses are listed in Appendix I.

How soon can I get a breast implant if I want one?

This is up to you. You might be able to have an implant at the same time as you have your original operation, or immediately after it. Some surgeons, however, still prefer to wait until it has been two years since the original operation. If this is not what you want, go back to your surgeon or to your family doctor and ask to have one sooner.

How will I ever feel able to start a new relationship?

Starting a new relationship after you have experienced physical changes to your body through cancer is not easy. When to tell and how much to say can put a great deal of pressure on you. Starting a new sexual relationship can feel almost impossible. Yet people **do** overcome their anxieties and fear of possible rejection and can have good, supportive relationships. As you come to terms with what has happened to you, both physically and emotionally, you are likely to find you gain in confidence which can help you to think about and perhaps try a new relationship.

There are always uncertainties with any new relationship. Having had cancer may add more, but it should not in itself stop you from beginning a new relationship. Besides, your new partner is just as likely to be anxious as you are and will be wondering what you think about them! This could far outweigh any concerns they have about you having had cancer.

Contraception and fertility

I've had cancer treatment. Can I still take the contraceptive pill?

This will depend on a number of factors, for example your age and the type of cancer and the treatment you have had. It may be advisable for you to change to another form of contraception, such as the sheath or coil.

Will taking the pill after having cancer increase the chances of another cancer developing?

It is possible that taking a contraceptive pill that has a high oestrogen content for several years may increase the chances of a young woman developing breast cancer later on. However, the majority of young women today are prescribed pills with a low oestrogen content. Research has shown that these may help to prevent cancer of the cervix and other gynaecological cancers.

Will having cancer affect my fertility?

The cancer might affect your fertility but it is more likely that the treatment could have this effect. Depending on the part of the body receiving treatment, surgery, chemotherapy and radio-therapy can all cause infertility, in both women and men, though in some cases this will be temporary. You should be warned before you have the treatment if this is a likely outcome.

It may be possible for a woman to have some ova (eggs) removed and frozen and stored before she starts any treatment and you should ask the hospital doctor if you want to find out more about this.

In men, the treatment might damage the sperm but not prevent its production. Damaged sperm can lead to genetic problems in children. It is advisable to wait at least a couple of years after treatment has finished and then to have your sperm tested before you attempt to father a child. It is sometimes possible to have your sperm banked before any treatment begins. You should check this out with the hospital doctors.

How soon after treatment is finished can I try to get pregnant?

That depends on the type of cancer and the treatment you have had and should be discussed with the hospital doctor. Some types of cancer are sensitive to hormone levels in the body. Pregnancy causes changes in your body's hormone levels, so the cancer might develop or come back. In general you should aim to wait for at least a couple of years before thinking about trying to conceive.

Can treatment bring on my menopause?

Having your ovaries removed surgically or having them irradiated can lead to an early menopause. You should be warned about this possibility before you have any treatment.

Employment

Should I tell my boss and my colleagues that I've got cancer?

That is entirely up to you. Some people tell everyone at work what is happening, some may tell only one or two people, and others choose not to tell anyone. You will probably need to provide some explanations if you are going to need to take time off or have to keep attending hospital appointments, but legally you do not have to tell your boss exactly what is wrong.

If you decide that you want someone at work to know about your cancer, but you want to be sure that the information remains confidential, it is worth remembering that occupational health staff are bound by confidentiality and cannot disclose medical details to your employer or anyone else without your permission.

Can I continue to work during my treatment?

If you feel able to continue to work then there is no reason to stop. Some radiotherapy treatment can lead to side effects which do not start to happen until the treatment is at least halfway through or even at its end. If you are having this type of treatment you might not initially need to take any time off except for hospital visits, but you might plan to have some time off later on.

Some people do not have side effects that affect them sufficiently to stop working during or after treatment, but you should consider not continuing to work if you are very tired or if it feels too much. A small amount of time off to recover is more likely to help you in the long term than sticking it out and ending up feeling considerably weaker for longer. Or you might find it helpful to work shorter hours or to take an occasional day off (for example, around the time you have chemotherapy) rather than stopping work all together.

Could I lose my job if I need to take time off work?

That depends on many things, particularly:

(i)   the type of contract you have, if any;
(ii) how long you have been working in your current position;
(iii) how much sick leave you have had in the current year;
(iv) your boss/employers;
(v)   how much time off you are taking.

If you have been working for the same employer for more than 16 hours a week in the same job for at least two years, you have certain employment rights (if less than 16 hours a week, you must have been with the same employer for five years). You can, however, be dismissed for taking long periods of time off sick if your employers have consulted with you about the time off and they could no longer reasonably be expected to keep the job open.

If you are a member of a trade union, you might find it helpful to talk to the union representative at work if you have any concerns about your employment rights.

Appendix II gives details of a booklet called **Cancer and Employment**.

I'm unemployed. Do I have to tell prospective employers that I have had cancer?

If you are asked about your health you should answer truthfully. If you don't and the truth comes out later on you run the risk of being dismissed no matter how long you have worked in the job or how well you carry out your work.

Will employers discriminate against me because I've had cancer?

It's possible. Any employer who operates an equal opportunities policy should not discriminate against any employee because they have or have had cancer. Such an employer is also unlikely to ask about your health record as part of any recruitment and selection process.

Many organisations and companies, however, do think twice about taking on a new member of staff who has had a serious illness of any kind. If you are asked you could present the truth in such a way as to try to allay some of the concerns the employer might have. For example, you could say that you have had treatment for cancer, that you continue to have regular check ups and that currently you are cancer-free, or that your cancer is being kept under control, according to which is the truth.

Often employers' prejudice is born out of ignorance. Many people still believe out-dated myths such as 'all cancer is incurable' or that 'cancer can be contagious'. More adults die of heart disease than of cancer in the UK and one of the most common causes of absenteeism from work is back problems, yet employees are not as likely to face discrimination on these grounds. If you do feel that you are being discriminated against because of your illness, and you are a member of a trade union, you should consult with your union representative.

With more people being successfully treated for cancer than ever before these attitudes are slowly starting to change. It does take time for people to recognise that the bad press cancer has had in the past does not necessarily apply today.

Going to college or university

Is there any point in going to college after I've had cancer?

This is a question that only you can answer. Some types of cancer have a very good prognosis (outlook) and some treatments have physical side effects which only last for a short time. Having cancer may make you want to rethink your future plans, and you may find you have different ideas now. Whether you are thinking about starting a college course, or whether you are already at college and have had to take time off because you have cancer, the decision could be made after you have spoken with various people:

(i)   the doctors who have been involved in your treatment;
(ii) a careers adviser at college or university;
(iii) a teacher;
(iv) a counsellor – many colleges employ counsellors for students;
(v)   a parent or guardian.

I've missed a term through having treatment. Is it better to go back or to wait and retake the whole year again?

Again, this is your decision. You might find it helpful to discuss various options that may be open to you with some of the people listed in the previous question. It could depend on how much work you have done (if any) while you have been off, and how you are feeling. It would be unwise to rush back into things and then find you have to take more time off because you are not yet well enough to cope with the workload. You might be able to go back part-time and to gradually ease yourself into the swing of things.

If you are receiving a grant, you may need to talk to someone to find out whether retaking a year will affect your entitlement.

Back to school

How can I help ease my child's return to school?

Keeping the teacher informed of what has been happening to your child and of how your child is feeling (both physically and emotionally) will enable the teacher to prepare the class for your child's return.

Many children worry about catching up with work they have missed. By asking the teacher to provide you with a regular programme of work for your child to do in hospital and at home, you can help to reduce some of the anxiety that a period of absence brings. You might want to ask the teacher to visit your child either in hospital or at home, or both. This can help your child to feel in touch with things.

Should the teacher tell the class what has been happening?

It is quite likely that the whole class will want to know how your child is, even if it is possible for some of them to visit. Often it is very helpful for the teacher to prepare the class for your child's return by telling them when she or he is coming back. The teacher can also pass on any special information, for example if your child won't be able to play outside at break times, or that your child might not look quite the same as before.

Your child might have her or his own views about what the class should be told, so you should check out what you were planning to say with her or him before any decisions are made between the teacher and yourself.

Some hospitals have play specialists who can come to the school with your child and explain to the rest of the class about the cancer and treatment that your child has had in a simple, clear and non-threatening way.

Appendix II gives information about **Welcome Back**, a booklet aimed at teachers concerned about a child returning to school after cancer treatment.

If someone in the class gets chickenpox, for example, should I keep my child off school?

Chickenpox is one of the most common viral infections of childhood and could be life-threatening if caught by a child who has cancer. A child who has recently had treatment for cancer or who is still having treatment may be able to continue to go to school even if there are these infections around, but it is best to check with the hospital doctor if you hear that a child in the class has got a viral infection. It may be possible to give your child a protective injection so that she or he can stay at school.

Finance

Where can I get some financial advice?

For more specific and detailed financial advice than is given here, you should speak to your personnel or welfare officer at work if there is one, or to the hospital social worker, or to your local **Citizens Advice Bureau** or **Benefits Agency** (Department of Social Security).

For more information about benefits and help if you are caring for an adult or a child who has cancer, you might find it useful to read leaflet FB31 **Caring for Someone** which you can get from your local Benefits Agency, post office or local advice agency. Some of the organisations listed in Appendix I may also be useful.

Am I entitled to sick pay if I can't work for a few months?

Each employer will have their own sick pay arrangements. Some only pay the legal minimum, while others are more generous. If you have been paying National Insurance contributions then you are likely to be able to receive either Statutory Sick Pay (SSP) or Sickness Benefit. They are both paid for up to a total of 28 weeks in any one financial year.

What happens if I'm off sick for longer than 28 weeks?

Your local Benefits Agency will usually transfer you to another longer term benefit which is called Invalidity Benefit.

Am I entitled to any other welfare benefits?

Your entitlement to welfare benefits depends on many factors and the benefits available change. For accurate, current information you should talk to someone who has detailed knowledge of the subject, such as the people and organisations suggested earlier in this section.

Can I claim benefits if I have to give up work or take a long time off to look after my child who has cancer?

In general, if you stop working voluntarily (that is to say, from choice), you are not eligible for welfare benefits. Individual employers may be willing to discuss ways in which you can take extended leave without losing your salary, or they may keep your job open for you for a period of time.

If you have not paid enough National Insurance contributions to ensure that you get a full pension, you may wish to protect your state pension if you are off work caring for a child or an adult who has cancer. In this case you could apply for Home Responsibilities Protection. Contact one of the organisations mentioned earlier in this section for more details.

Are there any organisations that can provide financial assistance for children who have cancer?

Yes, there are specialist funds available to provide financial support for children who have cancer in certain circumstances or for particular reasons. See Appendix I for more details.

Can I get life insurance if I have had cancer?

Different companies have different rules about this. Some companies will sell you life insurance if you have been disease free for a certain period of time and/or if your cancer was an early stage cancer. Other companies will only insure you for an extremely high premium, or will not consider insuring you at all, regardless of the type and stage of cancer.

You are unlikely to be able to get life insurance if it has been less than two years since you had cancer. Between two and seven years after having cancer some companies will insure you, but will probably charge a higher premium. If you are seven years cancer-and-recurrence-free, you will probably find you can get life insurance without incurring penalties.

Can I get a mortgage if I have had cancer?

You are likely to be able to get a mortgage even if it has been less than two years since you had cancer, but it will not have any life insurance cover (see previous question). The type and terms of the mortgage can sometimes depend on whether you are the sole person taking out the mortgage or if it is a joint one.

Can I get private medical cover if I have had cancer?

Most private medical insurance can be arranged so that it has certain exclusions, that is there will be situations in which you will not be able to claim. It is possible that if you have had cancer you will be able to have medical insurance but it may state that it will not pay out for anything to do with the cancer in the future. It is also possible that your premium will be increased once you have had cancer.

Practical help

I have a relative who has cancer. How can I be most helpful?

That depends on both of you, because what may be helpful for some may be anything but helpful for others. Relatives (and friends) often find it hard to know where to start to help the person who has cancer. A first step may be to ask what the person would find most helpful. Few of us wish to be a burden to our relatives and may not want to ask for 'a favour', but when help is offered we can sometimes find it easier to accept. It may be practical things like picking up children from school, helping to do the shopping, cooking a meal occasionally or going along for company when the person has hospital appointments. It may be being there at the end of a telephone at any time for a chat or perhaps phoning regularly yourself.

How do I get a wheelchair?

A wheelchair may be available for loan or hire from your local Red Cross Branch or from a local disability organisation. Social Services may be able to provide you with one on a permanent basis.

What about other aids?

Various aids are available from hospitals, from Social Services and from voluntary organisations. Assessments to see which aids might be helpful are done by occupational therapists who are either employed by the hospital or by the Social Services department.

How do I find out about getting adaptations made to my home?

An occupational therapist will make an assessment to see what might be useful. If you are being discharged from hospital, the hospital occupational therapist will do this. Otherwise there are occupational therapists who work for Social Services who can come and make the assessment. There may be a time lag between you putting in a request for an assessment and one actually taking place. It may be worth checking how long this might be at the outset, as you may need to arrange to borrow equipment in the meantime to help you to get by.

Am I being a nuisance if I ask for all these things?

No! It is very important to make sure that you have whatever you need to enable you to adapt your lifestyle to living with cancer.

7
The future . . .?

Introduction

Questions about the long term effects of cancer can be very difficult for someone to ask. Many of them are concerned with subjects which are rarely discussed - the possible recurrence of disease after treatment, living with incurable illness, or facing up to death. This chapter discusses all these questions, but also looks at the strengths that many people find as a result of having had cancer.

Is there a future after cancer?

Yes there is! In facing up to cancer, many people find they have strengths they might never have known about and discover things about themselves that they might never otherwise have had the chance to do. Having cancer can lead to people taking stock of their lives and making changes that they might never have dared to do.

That is not to underestimate the effects of cancer. For many people it is the worst and most devastating experience of their lives. Having to face up to things that few people would otherwise think about may cause emotional distress, psychological stress and have physical implications that could never have been imagined. Yet often, as time goes on, the initial shock waves subside and the side effects of treatment pass, and people are able to think once more about things other than their cancer.

Is it a good time to make changes?

Why not? For some people the enforced break in their regular routine that comes through having cancer is like being given a a chance to review things.

It can help you to realise that change is long overdue. Having had the courage to face your illness you may find that other changes are much less daunting. Perhaps you finally decide to stop doing something you've long since loathed and have done just for the sake of it. Perhaps you decide to make changes in your close relationships or work routine. Of course you are just as likely to acknowledge that you are quite satisfied with all aspects of your life.

Whatever the outcome of taking stock, many people come to view their cancer episode as a close shave that leads them to want to make the most of the future.

Recurrence

Will my cancer come back?

That is hard to answer. Some types of cancer are known to have a tendency to reappear some time later, perhaps in a different part of your body; other types are less likely to do this.

Even if the cancer you have had is one that is likely to recur, no one can tell you for certain when and how this might happen. And there will always be people who don't get a recurrence of their cancer, even though statistically this was thought to be likely.

Is it usual to worry that my cancer will come back?

The fear of having a recurrence of cancer is one that most people have. Often, the longer it is since you had the original cancer, the more the fear reduces, although it is not likely ever to go away completely. Some people say that the first thing they imagine whenever they have an ache or pain is that it is the cancer returning, even if logically they recognise this can not be the case.

What can I do to help myself when I think like this?

One thing you can do is to share your thoughts with someone so that you do not keep them bottled up inside, which allows the worry to build up and get quite out of proportion. You might find that someone who has had cancer would be a good person to talk to as it is likely they will have had similar feelings from time to time. This could be someone from a cancer support and self help group.

If you are worried that a cancer might be developing you can arrange to see the hospital doctor, by bringing your regular check up appointment forward if necessary.

I've had cancer. Does this mean that I could get another type in the future?

It is thought that there could be a slightly higher chance of getting a second, new cancer. However, having had cancer once, you will probably be having regular check ups. If you suspect anything could be developing, you can ask to see your hospital doctor between check ups and have any tests that are appropriate. This could mean that if you do have a new cancer, it can be treated at an early stage. In general, the earlier cancer is diagnosed, the more likely it is that it can be successfully treated.

What is a treatment-induced cancer?

Some treatments for cancer carry a small risk of leading to a new cancer in the future. This is a cancer that you wouldn't get if you had not had the original cancer and treatment.

How can I help myself to try to prevent getting another cancer?

By following the suggestions outlined in previous chapters about eating a balanced diet, reducing the amount you smoke (better still by stopping smoking), limiting the amount of alcohol you drink and taking regular exercise. All this will help to reduce the chances of a new cancer developing.

Why can no one be certain about my future?

One thing that everyone who has had cancer is wanting to hear is that their cancer is cured and that it will not come back. It is not usually possible to say this, except in a few specific cases. Although a great deal is known about many of the different types of cancer and their likely behaviour, cancer does not always follow the 'rules' – so no one is really able to provide a cast-iron guarantee that a cancer won't ever return.

Why do people talk about five and 10 year survival figures?

Researchers quote survival statistics, usually referring to people being free of cancer five or 10 years after it was diagnosed. These are only really of value for statistical purposes and to show possible trends in the population as a whole.

People who have cancer will often ask 'what are my chances?' but care should be taken when interpreting generalised statistics. If you are told that you have a 60% chance of being cancer-free in five years time, what does this really mean for you as an individual? Do you focus on this and ignore the other 40% chance? Or, if you are told you have a 40% chance of being alive and well in five years time, will you feel sure you will be amongst the 40% and not the other 60%? Remember statistics do not take into account each person's individual, specific situation.

There are times when I feel fine and then there are times when I am scared that I might die from my cancer. Is this common?

Yes, it is very common. Even several years after having cancer you may feel like this. This is something that relatives, friends and health professionals tend not to realise, particularly if it is some time since your treatment has finished, and this can make it hard to talk about your worries. Many people will have put your cancer experience to the back of their minds and may be surprised to hear you mention it, unless perhaps you are just about to go for a check up. It is really important that you do find someone to talk to about your feelings. You are not alone and there are many people who could identify with you and with your experience, but these may not be relatives or close friends. Appendix I lists organisations that can help you to find support.

What are metastases?

Metastases, which may be shortened to 'mets', is a word describing recurrent or secondary cancer. It means cancer that has spread from the original, or primary, cancer. The metastases could occur in another part of the body (distant metastases) or could be in the same place as before (local recurrence).

How do tests show that a cancer is a secondary rather than a primary cancer?

Cancer that has spread from one part of the body to another will contain cells that resemble and behave like those in the part of the body where the primary cancer was found. For example, under a microscope, cells from a breast cancer that has spread to a bone in the hip will look like breast tissue cells and they will behave like breast cancer, whereas the cells making up a primary bone cancer will look like bone cells and will behave like bone cancer.

Does it make any difference to the treatment if I have a recurrence of the original cancer or a new primary?

Yes, it does. The treatment may be quite different for a primary cancer than for a cancer which may develop in the same part of the body but which is a recurrence, or secondary, cancer. That is one of the reasons why it is very important to have tests done to establish which it is before embarking on a long course of treatment.

If my cancer does come back, can it be treated successfully?

That really depends on the type of cancer you had originally, where in the body it was and where it has reappeared. Successful treatment might mean the recurrence is removed from your body completely or it might mean that it is contained and prevented from spreading further.

Are the same options available for treating secondary cancer as there are for treating primary cancer?

Yes, it is possible to treat secondary cancer with one or more of surgery, radiotherapy, chemotherapy and hormone therapy.

Which may be most suitable for you will depend on several factors including:

(i)   the type of primary cancer;
(ii) how the primary cancer was treated;
(iii) where the secondaries are in your body;
(iv) how many secondaries there are.

Broadly speaking, chemotherapy and hormone therapy (which are treatments for the whole body) are more likely to be suggested if there are several metastases round the body or if this is thought to be something that could happen. Radiotherapy may be offered to you if you have a single metastasis or if you have a painful area due to a metastasis. Surgery can be used to remove a metastasis which may or may not be treated with one of the other options first, or surgery may be followed by one of the other types of treatment.

Is there a limit to how much treatment I can have?

Yes, but this depends on the type and quantity of treatment you have had already and to which parts of your body. For example, if you have had a high dose of radiotherapy to your chest, there will be a point at which you could not have any more radiotherapy in that area without causing permanent damage to the tissues. You could, however, have radiotherapy to another part of your body or you could have chemotherapy. So although there are limits, there are also choices.

What is palliation?

Palliation or palliative treatment is a term which describes the use of treatment to control or alleviate symptoms, such as pain, rather than to get rid of the cancer.

Does palliative treatment work?

Yes, some people live for a number of years having regular palliative treatment to keep symptoms at bay. Not being able to be cured does not mean that there is nothing that can be done to help you to continue to live as you would usually do.

I can't believe that it is not likely that my cancer could be cured. Isn't there something I can try that might still cure it?

When people are told that the treatment options are not likely to remove their cancer completely, many feel that there must be something new they could try which could provide them with renewed hope and a sense of not giving up. You should be very clear about your reasons for wanting to take action, whatever you decide to do, and you should be aware that it is possible that you may find that there is nothing that can help to remove your cancer. False hope can be more harmful in the long term than facing the hard news in the short term and finding a way of coping.

If you do decide you want to investigate other avenues there are a few ways in which you might proceed.

(i)   You might want to get a second opinion by going to see another specialist to see if another 'expert' has any alternative suggestions.

(ii) You might want to find out if anyone is carrying out a clinical trial into a particular type of treatment for the cancer you have.

(iii) Trying out certain complementary therapies might help you to feel as though you are continuing to do something active in terms of helping yourself and could provide long term benefits.

All these options are explained in more detail in previous chapters.

How long have I got to live?

This is one of the most common questions asked when a person is first told they have cancer or when they are told that the cancer is incurable. It is also almost impossible to answer. Some doctors feel they have to answer this question in some way rather than explaining why it is so difficult to answer. They may then say that a person has weeks rather than months to live or months rather than years. While it might be helpful to hear this, you should remember that one of the reasons a doctor could not be more precise is that cancer can be quite unpredictable. Even if you are told that you may live for several months, it is still possible you could be alive a few years later.

Terminal care and dying

What is terminal care?

Terminal care is the care of a dying person. It involves providing supportive treatment which takes account of all the person's needs. It enables the person to live a good quality of life until they die.

Good terminal care will ensure that someone does not suffer from unnecessary discomfort, that they receive adequate nutrition and that there is suitable equipment in the home to help their day-to-day routine. It also includes the use of suitable, effective painkillers as appropriate. It may involve some radiotherapy treatment as a means of controlling certain symptoms and may involve periods of time in a hospice.

A hospice is a place where you go to die, isn't it?

Hospices are places where people who are dying and those close to them can receive care and support in a number of ways. Some people feel confident and safe in a hospice and will choose to die there. Others prefer to die at home, and providing that the relatives or carers are properly supported by local health professionals, this can happen. In this case the hospice may be used for periods of respite care, to give both the person who is dying and their carers a break.

Why am I so scared of dying?

Nearly everybody is scared of dying. It is quite natural to be scared of something so final and so unknown. It can, nevertheless, be very helpful to try to work out what exactly your fears are, because some of them can possibly be lessened.

I'm scared about how I'm going to die. Will death be painful? Will I choke or bleed to death?

No one should die in pain as there are many types of pain relief, and a skilled health professional should be able to try different options to get one or several that are right for each individual. If you have pain that is not being controlled (and proper pain relief should not make you 'high', even if you are taking quite strong drugs), you should ask to see a specialist in pain and symptom control. Macmillan nurses and home care nurses are trained in symptom control, and they can spend time with you helping to find the right methods of pain relief for you. There are even 'pain clinics' in some parts of the country.

Although it is not possible to guarantee that you won't choke or bleed to death, very few people who are dying of cancer will die in this way.

Will I become incontinent?

The fear of losing control of your bladder or bowels is very common. It can happen. Aids such as catheters, special sheets to sit or lie on, and having a commode so that you don't have to worry about getting to the toilet can all help to ease the practical difficulties. With care and sensivitity from those who are caring for you, the embarrassment and loss of dignity that many people fear most can be reduced.

What happens to me after I die?

No one knows the answer to this question, and that is one reason why there are so many fears surrounding death. It is important that you share your feelings with someone. Voicing your thoughts means that you will not be carrying the burden of worry alone.

It is a sad fact that, for many of us, our culture does not permit us to talk openly about death. Yet if you can talk to someone (perhaps a person who is close to you or a professional counsellor), you are far more likely to be able to come to terms with your fears.

There are some things that you can choose to have happen after your death. For example, you can tell someone that you either want to be buried or to be cremated. You can choose the type of funeral service that you would like there to be. You can make a will to ensure that your possessions are handed down to those whom you would like to receive them.

Making a will and putting your affairs in order makes the practical things easier for the people that you leave behind. This can also give you the opportunity to think through the things you would like to do before you die, and the people to whom you would like to say goodbye.

What is a 'living will'?

A living will is a document which enables you to say what you would like to happen in the future, at a time when you may be too unwell to express an opinion. For example, you might not wish to have further treatment for your cancer or to have antibiotics or intravenous fluids. A living will is **not** a legal document. However, many doctors and your family and friends will probably take into account your wishes if you have considered carefully what might happen at that time, and have put your thoughts in writing. Organisations listed in Appendix I may be able to give you more information and advice about this.

Some days I feel so sad, other days I feel so angry and at other times I don't know what I feel. Why is this?

Coming to accept that you are dying is not something that happens overnight. Having to face your own death is bound to stir up all sorts of feelings and often you will have many different feelings at the same time. You may feel guilty, as though perhaps you are in some way to blame for not having fought hard enough or for getting cancer in the first place. You may feel angry that you are being cheated out of life. You will probably feel sad and need to grieve for what you will not be able to do.

It can help greatly if you are able to share your feelings with someone. You may need to cry for your sadness and for the losses you feel. Some people find that a relative, friend or a religious leader is the person they want to talk with. Others prefer to talk to someone who does not know them. Whichever you choose, talking and expressing the emotions you feel will help you to start to come to terms with what is happening.

Can I choose where I want to die?

To some extent, yes. Many people say they would prefer to die in their own homes, and with practical and emotional support for you and for the people caring for you, and with suitable medical support, this can be a good choice.

Other people prefer to die in a hospice. The atmosphere is usually one of peace and calm and the staff are very experienced in caring for those who are dying. Visitors are generally welcomed at any time. Some people go to a hospice for a short time (known as respite care), to give themselves and their carers a break – emotional as well as practical – returning home again a few days later.

Although there are hospices in most parts of the country, there are still places where this is not an option, but a local hospital may provide some respite care.

What if I try to care for my dying partner but it gets too much?

Anyone who is caring for a dying person at home needs support. As time goes on, it may become difficult for you to continue to care for your partner physically and emotionally. Many people underestimate the effect that caring for someone at home can have on them. If you find that it is getting too much it is really important to tell the health professionals (who should be visiting regularly) so that your partner can be moved into a hospice either on a temporary basis or permanently.

If you continue to struggle on it will become more and more difficult and you may lose out on the opportunity to spend valuable, good quality time with your partner.

But surely I should be able to manage to look after my partner on my own?

Caring for someone who is dying is extremely exhausting. Not only do you have to help physically, but you are also being emotionally affected by the situation. This adds to the weariness. Even if you have not been particularly close to each other, you are still going to be affected. It is important that you recognise when you have had enough and need to call on others, either in the short or long term.

Asking for help can relieve the strain and burden you are feeling. It does not mean that you have in any way failed. Rather, it is a very positive step to take because it can enable you to take some time for yourself, which can make you feel fresher and be of benefit to both of you.

It is my duty to care for a dying relative, isn't it?

There are people who believe they must take on this difficult task because it is expected of them. They may experience a sense of shame and guilt and failure if they do not. But there are many reasons why it may not be suitable for you to care for someone who is dying, one of the most important being that it is not what you want to do. It is hard to admit this in the face of pressure from those around us. Health professionals, too, may make assumptions about us that make it hard to say no.

But if you do not wish to take on this extremely difficult role, you must find a way of refusing. The dying person will probably sense that you are not comfortable in the role you have taken on, which can further add to the strain (although she or he may not say anything). Being a reluctant carer won't do either of you any good in the long run.

You might find it helpful to talk confidentially about the situation and your feelings to one of the cancer telephone information services listed in Appendix I.

If I want to get out of the house for a few hours – to do some shopping, for example – can I get someone to come in?

Yes, there are organisations which provide people who are able to come in for a few hours so that others in the household can go about doing other things. Night sitting services are also available to enable carers to sleep without having to be alert to the person's needs. These people might be trained care attendants or qualified nurses and the services are free. It is also possible to pay for private nursing cover. You may also be able to ask another relative or a friend to come in while you go out.

It is vital to take breaks away from the home and to get proper rest yourself when you are a carer. If at all possible, you should try to go out regularly, if only for a short time.

Will there be an increase in pain as death draws nearer?

No, this should not happen. It may be necessary to adjust the painkillers a person is taking or to try other techniques such as nerve blocks, but no one should have uncontrolled pain. Hospice staff have a great deal of experience in providing pain relief. Many hospices have home care nurses who will come to visit someone at home and who can adjust painkillers to provide greater relief if this is required. Macmillan nurses are also trained in pain control; they may be part of a home care team or may be hospital based.

How do you know that someone is about to die?

You may see a gradual deterioration over several days in the person's general condition. They may sleep for longer and longer periods of time. It is likely that they will not want to eat or drink much and may not want to get involved in what is going on around them. Some people also get a little confused. It is quite likely that a couple of days before someone dies their breathing will become shallower and there may be occasions when they seem to stop breathing for a short time. Periods of unconsciousness are also likely.

If death is expected, is it easier to cope with?

The death of someone you care about, even if it is expected, is still a shock. It is very important that you take care of yourself afterwards. You are not going to get through this difficult period more quickly just because you knew it was going to happen.

If you have had contact with a hospice, you will probably find you are offered the opportunity to talk to a bereavement counsellor who works there, or to join a bereavement support group based there. Throughout this book, talking to someone has been suggested as one thing that might be helpful, and it still applies now. See Appendix I for organisations that you might wish to contact to talk through your feelings after a death.

Although the second part of this chapter has been discussing aspects of terminal care and dying of cancer, it is worth remembering that one in three people who have cancer are treated successfully.

Appendix I

Useful organisations

The organisations listed here represent a range of national information sources and support networks for people affected by cancer. Local libraries and telephone directories may provide further information about regional or local sources of support.

The information listed is that provided by each organisation to the authors.

Cancer care and support

BACUP
3 Bath Place
Rivington Street
London EC2A 3JR
Tel: 0171 613 2121
Freephone: 0800 181199
Counselling Service: 0171 696 9000
Helps patients, their families and friends cope with cancer. Trained cancer nurses provide information, emotional support and practical advice by telephone or letter. A one-to-one counselling service is available, based at BACUP's office. Over 40 publications on cancer, its treatment and practical issues of coping.

Brain Tumour Foundation
PO Box 162
New Malden
Surrey KT3 3YN
Tel & Fax: 0181 336 2020
The organisation aims to increase awareness, throughout Great Britain, of the needs of individuals diagnosed with a brain tumour, and those of their families and significant others. To develop a support network, throughout Great Britain. To provide an educational and information resource for health

care professionals working in this field, survivors and their families about brain tumour disease, treatment, rehabilitation and support.

Breast Cancer Care
15-19 Britten Street
London SW3 3TZ
Helpline Tel: 0171 867 1103
Nationwide Freeline: 0500 245345

Edinburgh: Glasgow:
9 Castle Terrace   Suite 2/8
Edinburgh EH1 2DP   65 Bath Street, Glasgow G2 2BS
Helpline Tel: 0131 221 0407   Helpline Tel: 0141 353 1050
A free service of practical advice, information and support to women concerned about breast cancer. Volunteers who have had breast cancer themselves assist the staff in providing emotional support, nationwide.

British Colostomy Association
15 Station Road
Reading
Berkshire RG1 1LG
Tel: 0173 439 1537
An information and advisory service, giving comfort, reassurance and encouragement to patients to return to their previous active lifestyle. Emotional support is given on a personal and confidential basis by helpers who have long experience of living with a colostomy. Free leaflets and list of local contacts available. Can arrange visits in hospitals or at home on request.

British Red Cross Society
9 Grosvenor Crescent
London SW1X 7EJ
Tel: 0171 235 5454
The British Red Cross offers a range of services relevant to cancer patients, for example loan of wheelchairs, beauty care, and camouflage (on doctor's referral) and escort services to and from hospital. Please contact local branch or national headquarters for further details.

Cancer Care Society
21 Zetland Road
Redland
Bristol BS6 7AH
Tel: 0117 942 7419
Offers emotional support before, during and after treatment for patients and their families. A telephone link service allows people to talk to others in the same or similar circumstances. The counsellors offer personal and telephone support and there are support groups throughout the country.

CancerLink
17 Britannia Street
London WC1X 9JN
Tel: 0171 833 2451

Scotland:
9 Castle Terrace
Edinburgh EH1 2DP
Tel: 0131 228 5557

Asian Language Information and Support Line: 0171 713 7867
(Bengali, Hindi and English)
MAC Helpline for young people affected by cancer: 0800 591028
A textphone is available for people who are deaf or hard of hearing.

Provides emotional support and information on all aspects of cancer in response to letter and telephone enquiries from people with cancer, their families, friends and professionals working with them. Acts as a resource for over 500 cancer support and self help groups throughout the UK and helps people who set up new groups. Produces a range of publications on emotional and practical issues about cancer.

Cancer Relief Macmillan Fund
15/19 Britten Street
London SW3 3TZ
Tel: 0171 351 7811
Cancer Relief Macmillan Fund is a national charity, working to help improve the quality of life for people with cancer and their families. It funds the Macmillan Nursing Services, including Macmillan Paediatric Nurses, for home care and hospital support. The patient grants department provides financial help towards the cost of a wide range of things for people with cancer. Applications are made by a social worker, health visitor or community or home care nurse.

Cancer Research Campaign
10 Cambridge Terrace
London NW1 4JL
Tel: 0171 224 1333
The Cancer Research Campaign funds research into cancer ranging from prevention to cure. The research effort is complemented by an education programme.

Carers National Association
20-25 Glasshouse Yard
London EC1A 4JS
Carers Line Tel: 0171 490 8898
Other enquiries Tel: 0171 490 8818

Scotland:
11 Queen's Crescent
Glasgow G4 9AS
Tel: 0141 333 9495

Information and support to people who are caring at home. They also have a range of free leaflets. Branches and local offices throughout the country – for details of a local contact get in touch with the national office (address above).

Chai-Lifeline Cancer Support and Centre for Health
Norwood House
Harmony Way
off Victoria Road
London NW4 2BZ
Information Tel: 0181 202 2211
Helpline Tel: 0181 202 4567
Provides reassurance, support and friendship to Jewish cancer patients and their families, 24-hour telephone helpline, weekly support meetings, general information service, hospital and hospice visiting, spiritual guidance and public lectures. In addition, a wide range of complementary therapies are available for patients and well people together with wellbeing screening clinics for men and women.

Counsel and Care for the Elderly
Twyman House
16 Bonny Street
London NW1 9PG
Tel: 0171 485 1566 (Monday – Friday 10.30am – 4.00pm)
Advice service for old people, their relatives and professionals; information leaflets, grants to help people to remain in or return to their homes.

Crossroads Care Attendant Schemes
10 Regent Place
Rugby
Warwickshire CV21 2PN
Tel: 0178 857 3653
Provides care attendants who come into the home to give the carer a break. There are over 230 autonomous schemes throughout England, Scotland and Wales, with 10 regional offices.

CRUSE – Bereavement Care
Cruse House
126 Sheen Road
Richmond
Surrey TW9 1UR
Tel: 0181 940 4818
Cruse Bereavement Line: 0181 332 7227

Scotland:
18 South Trinity Road
Edinburgh EH5 3PN
Tel: 0131 551 1511

Wales:
Bryn Tirion
Churchill Close, Llanblethian
Cowbridge, S. Glamorgan CF7 7JH
Tel: 0144 677 5351

Cruse offers a comprehensive service of counselling by trained and selected people, advice on practical matters and opportunities for social support. This service is available to all bereaved people either through one of its 192 branches or national membership. There is a wide range of supportive, informative and advisory literature and a monthly magazine. In addition Cruse arranges training courses for those who work either in a professional or lay capacity with the bereaved.

DIAL UK (Disablement Information and Advice Lines)
Park Lodge
St Catherine's Hospital
Tickhill Road
Balby
Doncaster DN4 8QN
Tel: 0130 231 0123
DIAL UK is the national association for the DIAL network of over 100 disability information and advice services. DIAL groups give free, independent and impartial advice on all aspects of disability. They are run and staffed by people with direct experience of disability.

Disabled Living Foundation
380–384 Harrow Road
London W9 2HU
Tel: 0171 289 6111
Fax: 0171 266 2922
National resource for information about equipment to help people with a disability carry out daily living activities.

Disability Scotland
Princes House
5 Shandwick Place
Edinburgh EH2 4RG
Phone & Minicom: 0131 229 8632
Fax: 0131 229 5168
National resource (Scotland only) for information on aids and equipment for people with a disability.

Family Health Services Authority
Look in the phone book under Family Health Service Authority or in Yellow Pages under **Health Authorities and Services**. (The name changed in 1990 from Family Practitioner Committee.)

GEMMA
BM Box 5700
London WC1N 3XX
Tel: 0171 485 4024
A national self help group of lesbians and bisexual women with or without disabilities. Formed in 1978 to lessen the isolation of disabled lesbians. Issue a quarterly newsletter, in print and on tape.

Hodgkin's Disease and Lymphoma Association
PO Box 275
Haddenham
Aylesbury
Bucks HP17 8JJ
Helpline: 0184 429 1500 (9.00am–10.00pm 7 days a week)
Office: 0184 429 1479 (9.00am–5.00pm Monday – Friday)
We provide emotional support and information for lymphoma (Hodgkin's disease and non-Hodgkin's lymphoma) patients and their families. Literature and videos available. Quarterly newsletter. National network of helpers with experience of the disease, with whom enquirers may be linked, usually by telephone. Local groups in some areas.

Holiday Care Service
2 Old Bank Chambers
Station Road
Horley
Surrey RH6 9HW
Tel: 0129 377 4535
Minicom: 0129 377 6943
Fax: 0129 378 4647
Advice and information on holidays and travel arrangements for people who are disabled or elderly.

Hospice Information Service
St Christopher's Hospice
51–59 Lawrie Park Road
Sydenham
London SE26 6DZ
Tel: 0181 778 9252
The Hospice Information Service publishes a directory of hospice services which provides details of hospices, home care teams, and hospital support teams in the UK and the Republic of Ireland. For copies of the directory or details of local services, including hospice services for children, write or telephone.

Hysterectomy Support Network
3 Lynne Close
Green Street Green
Orpington
Kent BR6 6BS
'New Horizon' booklet: £1.50
Annual Membership – £6.00 (waged) £3.50 (unwaged)
Write direct for information enclosing SAE.

ia Ileostomy and Internal Pouch Support Group
Amblehurst House
PO Box 23
Mansfield
Notts NG18 4TT
Tel & Fax: 01623 28099
ia offers a wide range of advisory services through local groups and national advisers. If you write to the association and require a reply, please include a large stamped, self-addressed envelope.

Impotence Information Centre
PO Box 1130
London W3 9BB
An information centre providing literature relating to impotence, causes and treatments. Mailing service only.

Irish Cancer Society
5 Northumberland Road
Dublin 4
Republic of Ireland
Tel: 010353 1 6681855
Fax: 010353 1 6687599
Freephone in Republic of Ireland 1800 200 300
The Irish Cancer Society is the national charity dedicated to preventing cancer, saving lives from cancer and improving the quality of life of those living with cancer, through care, education and research. Lectures and talks are provided to the workplace, schools, public and professional organisations. Range of literature – posters are available on the Cancer Helpline – to discuss personal enquiries on the free telephone.

Lesbian Network
c/o CancerLink
17 Britannia Street
London WC1X 9JN
Phone & Textphone: 0171 833 2451
The network provides an opportunity for lesbians affected by cancer to give and receive support.

Lesbian & Gay Bereavement Project
Vaughan Williams Centre
Colindale Hospital
London NW9 5HG
Helpline Tel: 0181 455 8894
A recording gives number for member on duty that evening. Telephone helpline for people bereaved by the death of a same-sex partner. Also offers a free will form and notes in return for an SAE. As well as giving telephone advice and support project members can speak on same-sex loss to nurses, social workers and others concerned with death and dying.

Let's Face It
10 Wood End
Crowthorne
Berkshire RG11 6DQ
Tel: 0134 477 4405
Let's Face It is an international mutual help organisation dealing with facial disfigurement. It is dedicated to helping those who are facially disfigured, their loved ones, the professionals who care for them and the communities in which they live, to understand and solve the problems of living with this disability.

Leukaemia Care Society
14 Kingfisher Court
Venny Bridge
Pinhoe
Exeter, Devon EX4 8JN
Tel: 0139 246 4848
The Leukaemia Care Society aims to promote the welfare of those persons (and their families) suffering from leukaemia and allied blood disorders. It offers support, friendship, information leaflets, financial assistance and caravan holidays.

Leukaemia Research Fund
43 Great Ormond Street
London WC1N 3JJ
Tel: 0171 405 0101
Publishes informative booklets for people with leukaemia and their families.

Lymphoedema Support Network
c/o The Appeal Office
Royal Marsden NHS Trust
Fulham Road
London SW3 6JJ
Tel: 0171 433 3410 or 0181 748 2403
The Lymphoedema Support Network is a small charity run by volunteer patients with lymphoedema, offering bi-annual newsletters, information, practical advice and support to all lymphoedema patients.

Mind Over Matter
14 Blighmont Crescent
Millbrook
Southampton
Hampshire SO15 8RH
Tel: 0170 377 5611 (ansaphone)
Meeting Place: Southampton
A voluntary group set up to increase men's awareness of testicular cancer. Offers individual befriending for patients and their families, through tele-

phone counselling with home and hospital visits where appropriate. Meetings are held informally in a relaxed environment for emotional support.

Marie Curie Cancer Care
28 Belgrave Square
London SW1X 8QG
Tel: 0171 235 3325
Marie Curie Cancer Care provides nursing care for people with cancer, through 11 in-patient Marie Curie Centres. Over 4,500 Marie Curie nurses nationwide are available to nurse patients in their own homes. All services to patients are free of charge. Marie Curie Cancer Care also runs its own Research Institute and the Education Department provides training courses and conferences for health professionals on cancer and related topics.

National Association of Bereavement Services
20 Norton Folgate
London E1 6DB
Referrals: 0171 247 1080
Fax/Admin: 0171 247 0617
A support organisation for bereavement services, making referrals nationally to the most local of the specialised services needed.

National Association of Citizens Advice Bureaux
115–123 Pentonville Road   Scotland:
London N1 9LZ   26 George Square
Tel: 0171 833 2181   Edinburgh EH8 9LD
                                 Tel: 0131 667 0156

North Wales: South Wales:
134b High Street   Andrews Buildings
Prestatyn   67 Queen Street
Clwyd LL19 9BN   Cardiff CF1 4AW
Tel: 0174 585 6339   Tel: 0122 239 7686
Local advice centres throughout the country.

National Association of Laryngectomee Clubs
Ground Floor
6 Rickett Street
London SW6 1RU
Tel: 0171 381 9993
Promote the welfare of laryngectomees within the British Isles. Encourages the formation of clubs with objective of assisting rehabilitation through speech therapy, social support and monthly meetings. Advises on speech aids and medical supplies. Offers referral service.

National Cancer Alliance
PO Box 579
Oxford OX4 1LP
Tel: 0186 579 3566

A new voluntary organisation of patients and health care professionals formed to voice the concerns and opinions of people affected by cancer about the services, care and treatment provided. Information, education and advice about good care and services and what standards of care and treatment people have a right to expect, how to get it and how to provide it.

Oesophageal Patient's Association
16 Whitefields Crescent
Solihull
West Midlands B91 3NU
Tel: 0121 704 9860
Leaflets, telephone advice and support, before and during treatment. Visits, where possible, by former patients to people with oesophageal cancer.

Patients Association
18 Victoria Park Square
Bethnal Green
London E2 9PF
Tel: 0181 981 5676
The Patients Association is an independent organisation offering advice to patients and representing their interests. The Association produces information leaflets and a directory of self help health organisations and will answer queries by letter or telephone on health service or private medicine problems.

Royal Association for Disability & Rehabilitation (RADAR)
12 City Forum
250 City Road
London EC1V 8AF
Tel: 0171 250 3222
Minicom: 0171 250 0212
Campaigning and advisory body in the field of physical disability, producing a large number of publications on areas such as holidays, mobility, leisure, education, employment and rights.

Save Our Sons
Tides Reach
1 Kite Hill
Wootton Bridge
Isle of Wight PO33 4LA
Tel: 0198 388 2876
Testicular cancer information service, giving help and advice over the telephone – after 5pm if possible. Also publicises the need for testicular self-examination. Leaflet on testicular self-examination (SAE please).

Society for the Prevention of Asbestosis and Industrial Diseases
38 Drapers Road
Enfield
Middlesex EN2 8LU
Tel: 01707 873025
Encourages research into the causes, prevention and treatment of asbestosis and other industrial diseases. Provides information and advice for those who become ill or disabled through industrial disease; collates information about causes and works for prevention.

SPOD
(Association to aid the Sexual and Personal Relationships of People with a Disability)
286 Camden Road
London N7 0BJ
Tel: 0171 607 8851
Provides information and advice on problems in sex and personal relationships which disability can cause. General leaflets and reading lists available, and individual advice given on request. Publications list available.

Tak Tent Cancer Support – Scotland
The Western Infirmary
Block C20
Western Court
100 University Place
Glasgow G12 6SQ
Tel: 0141 211 1932 (Resource Centre)
Tel: 0141 211 1931 (Appeals)
Offers information, support, education and care for cancer patients, families, friends and health professionals. Network of support groups across Scotland, meeting monthly in the evening. 'Drop In' Resource and Information Centre now open.

Tenovus Cancer Information Centre
PO Box 88
College Buildings
Courtenay Road
Splott
Cardiff CF1 1SA
Tel: 0122 249 7700
Freephone Helpline: 0800 526527
Fax: 0122 248 9919
Although the primary concern is prevention, the Centre provides information and advice on all cancer-related concerns. Contact by telephone, letter or personal visit.

Urostomy Association (Central Office)
'Buckland', Beaumont Park
Danbury
Essex CM3 4DE
Tel & Fax: 0124 522 4294
Assists patients both before and after surgery for the removal of the bladder and advises on appliances, housing, work situation or marital problems and helps them to resume as full a life as possible with confidence. 27 regional branches hold meetings on a regular basis. Will arrange hospital and home visits on request.

Ulster Cancer Foundation
Cancer Information Service
40/42 Eglantine Avenue
Belfast BT9 6DX
Tel: 0123 266 3281
Involved in many aspects of cancer, from prevention to patient support. Operates an information helpline for cancer-related queries for patients and their families, staffed by experienced cancer nurses, who can arrange counselling by personal appointment at the centre.

Women's Health
52 Featherstone Street
London EC1Y 8RT
Tel: 0171 251 6580
Information on women's health available to all women; works for improvements in women's health services. Library and information service centre for women's groups. Produces excellent information sheets. List available.

Women's Health Concern
83 Earls Court Road
London W8 6EF
Tel: 0171 938 3932
Fax: 0171 376 0879
WHC's main aim is to provide medical information about the menopause and to advise doctors and women about the appropriate use of HRT. The charity helps women with gynaecological, hormonal and other women's health problems. It provides publications, counselling, and postgraduate symposia and training courses for doctors and nurses. Counselling services available in some areas, contact office for further details.

Women's Nationwide Cancer Control Campaign
Suna House
128-130 Curtain Road
London EC2 3AR
Tel: 0171 729 4688
Helpline Tel: 0171 729 2229

Encourages measures for the prevention and early detection of cancer in women. Produces a wide range of leaflets, posters.

Complementary care

British Holistic Medical Association
179 Gloucester Place
London NW1 6DX
Tel: 0171 262 5299
Aims to educate doctors and other health care professionals so that patients are treated as individuals. Publishes a quarterly newsletter for members, also self help cassettes and books. Send SAE for publications list.

Cancer Help Centre
Grove House
Cornwallis Grove
Clifton
Bristol BS8 4PG
Tel: 0117 974 3216
The Centre aims to meet the needs of cancer patients and their families by offering a holistic approach to help with the physical, emotional, psychological and spiritual problems experienced by people diagnosed as having cancer.

Community Health Foundation
188 Old Street
London EC1V 9FR
Tel: 0171 251 4076
Please write to the above for further information about the macrobiotic diet and meditation.

Hospice Arts
Forbes House
9 Artillery Lane
London E1 7LP
Tel: 0171 377 8484
Hospice Arts' prime objective is to develop and encourage the range of creative arts opportunities for hospice patients. Offers advice and support to hospice arts projects and will advise on potential sources of funding. It also evaluates projects and organises training sessions.

Institute for Complementary Medicine
PO Box 194
London SE16 1QZ
Tel: 0171 237 5165
Runs the British Register of Complementary Practitioners and can supply names of reliable practitioners of various kinds of complementary medicine, such as homeopathy, relaxation techniques, and osteopathy. Also has contact with other support groups. Please send SAE for information, stating area of interest.

New Approaches to Cancer
5 Larksfield
Egham
Surrey TW20 0RB
Tel: 0178 443 3610
A charity which promotes the holistic attitude to cancer, through a positive attitude to self help. Local groups throughout the UK.

Acupuncture
British Acupuncture Association and Register
34 Alderney Street
London SW1V 4EU
Tel: 0171 834 1012
Can supply, for a fee of £2.50, a register of members which includes many trained practitioners with additional medical knowledge and/or qualifications.

British Medical Acupuncture Society
Newton House
Newton Lane
Whitley
Warrington WA4 4JA
Tel: 0192 573 0727
Promotes the use and understanding of acupuncture as part of the practice of medicine. Trains qualified doctors and dentists. Publishes a journal. A list of members and a patient information leaflet is available to the public.

Art therapy
British Association of Art Therapists
11a Richmond Road
Brighton
Sussex BN2 3RL
Tel: 0173 426 5407
Fax: 0127 368 5852
Provides information, for a fee, about training courses for art therapy and maintains a register of practising art therapists.

Person-centred Art Therapy Association
115 High Street
Lewes
East Sussex BN7 1XY
Tel: 0127 347 4505
Enables people who believe in bringing together the person-centred counselling approach with art therapy to share ideas and practices.

Counselling
British Association for Counselling
1 Regent Place
Rugby
Warwickshire CV21 2PJ
Tel: 0178 857 8328
Provides list of counsellors divided into counties, giving counsellor's qualifications, type of problems counselled and probable cost; and information sheet with counselling guidelines.

Healing
Churches Council for Health and Healing
St Marylebone Parish Church
Marylebone Road
London NW1 5LT
Tel: 0171 486 9644
Puts people in touch with churches in their area involved with the ministry of Christian healing. A 24-hour answerphone service is available.

Confederation of Healing Organisations
Suite J, Second Floor
The Red & White House
113 High Street
Berkhamsted, Hertfordshire HP4 2DJ
Tel: 0144 287 0660
Advice, Messages and Fax: 0144 287 0660
The Confederation of Healing Organisations provides contact and distant healing from its 12 member associations with 6200 healers in the UK. All are regulated by the same compulsory Code and Disciplinary Procedures, covered by public liability and professional indemnity insurance comparable to a GP's and accept the same minimum criteria for entry and training. Access to a healer may be had from the NFSH (0189 161 6080) and BAHA (0122 737 3804) or for more information via CHO's Head Office. No belief is required of patients. Fees, if any, are moderate. The Department of Health has advised that their Patients' Charter entitles patients wishing to see a healer to request this in NHS hospitals.

National Federation of Spiritual Healers
Old Manor Farm Studio
Church Street
Sunbury-on-Thames
Middlesex TW16 6RG
Tel: 0193 278 3164
Referrals only: 0189 161 6080
Fax: 0193 277 9648
Maintains a list of member healers in all parts of the UK. Expect a four week delay in replies, except in emergency cases. Healers are allowed to visit and

treat patients in NHS hospitals (must be invited by patients and must not discuss medical treatments).

Herbalism
British Herbal Medicine Association
Sun House
Church Street
Stroud
Gloucestershire GL5 1SL
Tel: 0145 375 1389
Contact for a list of practitioners within your local area.

National Institute of Medical Herbalists
9 Palace Gate
Exeter EX1 1JA
Tel: 0139 242 6022
Written and telephone enquires for practitioner in your local area and for information on herbalism.

Homoeopathy
British Homoeopathic Association
27a Devonshire Street
London W1N 1RJ
Tel: 0171 935 2163
The Association has a list of all homoeopathic doctors and hospitals throughout the UK and has a lending library for members. Publishes a bi-monthly journal and has leaflets on homoeopathy.

Society of Homoeopaths
2 Artizan Road
Northampton
NN1 4HU
Tel: 01604 21400
The Society publishes a Register of professional homoeopaths in the UK as well as information leaflets. Register and leaflets are available free of charge on receipt of a large self-addressed envelope.

Massage: aromatherapy
International Federation of Aromatherapists
Stamford House
2–4 Chiswick High Road
London W4 1TH
Tel: 0181 742 2605
Written enquiries only enclosing SAE.

International Society of Professional Aromatherapists
Hinckley & District Hospital & Health Care Centre
The Annex
Mount Road
Hinckley
Leicestershire LE10 1AG
Tel: 0145 563 7987
Fax: 0145 589 0956
Write for list of practitioners within your local area.

Massage: reflexology
Association of Reflexologists
27 Old Gloucester Street
London WC1N 3XX
Information may be obtained by writing to the above address or by contacting
Mr G. Woodward (Administrator) on Tel: 0127 347 9020

British Reflexology Association
Monks Orchard
Whitbourne
Worcester WR6 5RB
Tel: 0188 682 1207
An ancient therapy in which feet – and more rarely palms of hands – are
treated by a pressure point technique. Register of members available (£1.50)
and details of reflexology training courses, books and charts can be supplied.

Relaxation
Relaxation for Living
168–170 Oatlands Drive
Weybridge
Surrey KT13 9ET
Tel: 0193 283 1000
Promotes the teaching of physical relaxation. Holds small group classes
around the UK and runs a correspondence course for pupils out of reach of a
teacher. Publishes self help tapes and leaflets. Runs regular courses for
relaxation teachers. Send a large stamped addressed envelope for
information.

Yoga
British Wheel of Yoga
1 Hamilton Place
Boston Road
Sleaford
Lincs NG34 7ES
Encouragement and help for people to understand all aspects of yoga and its
practice; maintains standards of yoga teaching; organises and supports local
branches; publications list available.

Support for children and their families

ACT (Association for Children with life-threatening or Terminal conditions & their families)
65 St Michael's Hill
Bristol BS2 8DZ
Tel: 0117 922 1556
Aims to make information available to all parents and professionals about support services for families throughout the country, both statutory, voluntary and self-help groups. Will respond to telephone and written enquiries, and also assist in the development of new services by bringing together, in informal meetings, people with appropriate ideas and expertise.

Action for Sick Children (National Association for the Welfare of Children in Hospital)
Argyle House
29/31 Euston Road
London NW1 2SD
Tel: 0171 833 2041
Provides an information, advice and support service, conferences, reports and publications for parents and children and health professionals.

Action for Sick Children (Scotland)
15 Smith's Place
Edinburgh EH6 8TN
Tel: 0131 553 6553
Action for Sick Children (Scotland) has 11 local groups throughout Scotland. They: (i) support sick children and their families; (ii) ensure that parents have unrestricted access to their children in hospital; (iii) work to improve services for sick children and facilities for parents in hospital; (iv) provide information about hospital for children and parents, and lend hospital playboxes to pre-5 groups and primary schools.

CALL (Childhood Cancer and Leukaemia Link)
36 Knowles Avenue
Crowthorne
Berkshire RG11 4DU
Tel: 0134 475 0319
Aims to provide understanding, support and information for families. Links families in a similar area or situation who are kept in touch nationally via a quarterly newsletter. Some social activities and meetings. Annual parents day and Easter party. Will pray for families if requested.

Children's Cancer Support Group (CHICS)
88 Vaughan Road
Wallasey
Wirral L45 1LP

Information available on other groups. Group provides an informal forum where patients can share their experiences, problems and emotions and can receive information and support. Provides link-ups with other organisations. Organises social events and outings, arranges ward coffee evenings. Produces a newsletter.

Children's Trust
Tadworth Court
Tadworth
Surrey KT20 5RU
Tel: 0173 735 7171
Services for chronically sick and disabled children. Short term respite care.

Christian Lewis Trust
Child Care Centre
62 Walter Road
Swansea SA1 2JQ
Tel: 0179 248 0500
Tel: Careline 0179 248 0600
Our Mission Statement 'Caring for children with cancer' covers all children and teenagers with any form of cancer and whatever stage they are at with their treatment. We provide understanding, encouragement and positive caring support in various ways. Our national telephone Careline offers a confidential 'listening ear' for anyone whose life is, or ever has been, affected in any way by a child with cancer. We also provide crisis breaks, at our two holiday sites in Wales; specialised travel insurance schemes; welfare grants; bereavement support; befriending by letter; quarterly newsletter. Locally our care and support is offered on a face to face basis and through monthly support group meetings. Our children's cancer continuing care nurses and play therapist work directly with children and their families in their homes as well as liaising with the local health authorities.

Cancer and Leukaemia In Childhood
CLIC House
11/12 Fremantle Square
Cotham, Bristol BS6 5TL
Tel & Fax: 0117 924 4333
CLIC offers help to children with cancer or leukaemia and their families through a well-established 'model of care' including home-care nursing, individual financial assistance, special holidays and 'home-from-home' family accommodation.

Compassionate Friends
53 North Street
Bristol BS3 1EN
Tel: 0117 953 9639
Fax: 0117 966 5202

A nationwide self help organisation of parents whose child of any age, including adult, has died from any cause. Personal and group support. A quarterly newsletter, a postal library and a range of leaflets. A befriending, not counselling, system. Works through a system of county contacts and group leaders, located throughout the country.

Contact A Family
170 Tottenham Court Road
London W1P 0HA
Tel: 0171 383 3555
Fax: 0171 383 0259
Network of support groups for parents of children with special needs and disabilities. Information and advice line plus specialist groups for rare syndromes and genetic conditions. Over 1000 local support groups and 500 national bodies.

Edward's Trust
87 Stirling Road
Edgbaston
Birmingham B16 9BD
Tel: 0121 455 6257
To provide accommodation, information, assistance and support to families and friends of children with cancer and to increase awareness of all approaches to the disease.

Institute of Family Therapy
43 New Cavendish Street
London W1M 7RG
Tel: 0171 935 1651
Fax: 0171 224 3291
The Institute's Elizabeth Raven Memorial Fund offers free counselling to families who have suffered a bereavement within the past 12 months, or those with seriously ill family members. Works with the whole family. While the service is free, voluntary donations to the fund are accepted to help other families.

Make a Wish Foundation UK
Suite B, Rossmore House
26-42 Park Street
Camberley
Surrey GU15 3PL
Tel: 01276 24127
Will grant the favourite wish of a child aged between 3-18 years who is suffering from a life-threatening illness.

Malcolm Sargent Cancer Fund for Children
14 Abingdon Road
London W8 6AF
Tel: 0171 937 4548
Fax: 0171 376 1193
Aims to help all young people under 21 years who have any form of cancer –
either in their homes or in hospital. It is a welfare organisation – not research.
Funds Malcolm Sargent social workers in the major paediatric oncology
centres throughout the British Isles. Also owns two holiday homes and
sponsors Malcolm Sargent camps on Lake Windermere.

NASPCS – The Charity for Incontinent and Stoma Children
51 Anderson Drive
Valley View Park
Darvel
Ayrshire KA17 0DE
Tel: 0156 032 2024
To provide a contact and information service for parents on the practical day
to day management of all aspect of coping with a child with either a
colostomy, ileostomy or urostomy. Also gives advice on the incontinence often
encountered with bowel and bladder problems.

National Holiday Fund for Sick & Disabled Children
Suite 1, Princess House
1-2 Princess Parade
New Road
Dagenham
Essex RM10 9LS
Tel: 0181 595 9624
Fax: 0181 593 8755
Aims to relieve the sickness of the chronically or terminally ill children
between 8-18 years old by providing holidays at selected venues throughout
the world.

Neuroblastoma Society
41 Towncourt Crescent
Petts Wood
Kent BR5 1PH
Tel & Fax: 0168 987 3338
Information and advice by telephone or letter for patients and their families.
Provides contact where possible with others who have experienced the illness
in the family, for mutual support.

Rainbow Centre for Children with Cancer and Life-Threatening Illness
PO Box 604
Bristol BS99 1SW
Tel: 0117 973 0752 or 0117 973 6228 (24hr ansaphone)

Offers therapeutic support and complementary therapies, which may be used alongside any other treatment. Support given to the sick child and his or her parents, brothers and sisters, and the family as a whole. Also available to anyone who needs support and space to grieve after a child's death. Visualisation/relaxation/meditation. Help with diet, vitamin and mineral supplements.

Retinoblastoma Society
c/o Academic Department of Paediatric Oncology
St Bartholomew's Hospital
West Smithfield, London EC1A 7BE
Tel: 0171 600 3309 (ansaphone)
Links familes in the same situation and area, to give moral support and practical help. Creates an opportunity for parents to exchange information and share experiences. Distribution of newsletter 2–3 times per year with contributions from parents and professionals.

United Kingdom Children's Cancer Study Group (UKCCSG)
Department of Epidemiology & Public Health
University of Leicester
Clinical Services Building
Leicester Royal Infirmary
PO Box 65
Leicester LE2 7LX
Tel: 0116 252 3280
Fax: 0116 252 3281
The UKCCSG co-ordinates the management, in all its aspects, of the majority of children with cancer in the United Kingdom (excluding leukaemia). Provides an information booklet for the parents of children with cancer.

Appendix II

Useful publications

There are now several books available about cancer and its treatment, and many more on complementary therapy or ways of reducing stress and increasing well-being. A browse through the health section of a large bookshop or your local library will help you to select a book which suits you. The following titles have been chosen as examples of what is available. Where a title has been mentioned in the book, it is marked with an *.

The Health Care Consumer Guide   Robert Gann
Faber & Faber, 1991

Cancer: A Guide for Patients and   Chris & Sue Williams
   their Families   John Wiley, 1988
(Originally written in 1986, this is still a good basic guide although many changes have taken place regarding treatment)

Bowel Cancer: The Facts   J. Northover & J. Kettner
Oxford University Press, 1992

Breast Cancer: A Guide for Every   M. Baum, C. Saunders &
   Woman   S. Meredith
Oxford Medical Publications, 1994

Lung Cancer: The Facts   C. Williams
Oxford University Press, 1992

Facing Death   Averil Stedeford
William Heineman Medical Books, 1985

When your Mum or Dad has Cancer   Ann Couldrick
Sobell Publications, 1991

I Don't Know What to Say   R. Buckman
Papermac, 1988

I Can Cope: Staying Healthy with Cancer	J. Johnson & L. Klein Chronimed, 1994
Recipes for Health: Cancer	C. Shaw & M. Hunter Thorsons, 2nd edition, 1995
Wells' Supportive Therapies in Health Care	R. Wells & V. Tschudin Balliere Tindall, 1994

(Although written for health professionals, this book is also accessible to the general reader)

Complementary Care and Cancer	CancerLink 2nd edition, 1993
* Cancer and Employment	CancerLink, 1992
* Lymphoedema – Advice on Treatment	C. Regnard, C. Badger & P. Mortimer Beaconsfield Publishers, 2nd edition, 1991
* The Householders' Guide to Radon	Department of the Environment, 3rd edition, 1991 2 Marsham Street London SW1P 3EB

Booklets and leaflets

The **Royal Marsden NHS Trust** has a series of booklets in their **Patient Information Series**. Each booklet focuses on a specific cancer, test, treatment or side effect. Titles include ***Breast Reconstruction**, ***Clinical Trials** and ***Laryngectomy**. A complete list of the titles available (33 in total) can be obtained from:
Haigh and Hochland Publications
174A Ashley Road
Hale
Cheshire WA15 9SF
Tel: 0161 929 0190
Fax: 0161 929 1818

CancerLink produces booklets which focus on the psychological and emotional aspects of coping with cancer. A full publications list is available from CancerLink (address in Appendix I).

BACUP produces booklets in a series called **Understanding Cancer**. These cover many types of cancer and their treatments. A full publications list is available from BACUP (address in Appendix I).

Breast Cancer Care produces a number of leaflets and booklets that cover different aspects of living with breast surgery. A full publications list is available from BCC (address in Appendix I).

The **Cancer Research Campaign** has a number of booklets and factsheets. Titles include **Skin Cancer, the Sun and You*, and **Welcome Back! How teachers can help children returning to school after treatment for cancer*. A full list of publications is available from The Education Department of the Cancer Research Campaign (address in Appendix I).

The **Hodgkin's Disease and Lymphoma Association** (HDLA) produces booklets and leaflets that are concerned with living with lymphomas. Details are available from HDLA (address in Appendix I).

The **National Association for Mental Health** (MIND) produces a number of booklets, some of which are concerned with coping with caring, depression and bereavement. A full publications list can be obtained from:
MIND Publications
Granta House
15-19 Broadway
Stratford
London E15 4BQ
Tel: 0181 519 2122

The **Hodgkin's Disease Association** (HDA) produces booklets and leaflets that are concerned with living with lymphomas. Details are available from HDA (address in Appendix I).

The **National Association for Mental Health** (MIND) produces a number of booklets, some of which are concerned with coping with caring, depression and bereavement. A full publications list can be obtained from:

MIND Publications Mail Order Service
4th Floor
24–32 Stephenson Way
London NW1 2HD
Tel: 071-387 9126

Index

Have you found **Cancer information at your fingertips** practical and useful? If so, you may be interested in other books in this ". . . *at your fingertips*" series from Class Publishing.

Asthma at your fingertips
REVISED EDITION
Dr Mark Levy, Professor Sean Hilton and Sister Greta Barnes

The more you understand your asthma, the better you can manage it and keep it under good control – and good management makes it easier to live a full, happy and healthy life.

> "Having asthma should not stop you leading a full and active life . . . This book gives you the knowledge. Don't limit yourself."
> *Adrian Moorhouse, MBE, Olympic Gold Medallist*

Allergies at your fingertips
Dr Joanne Clough and Dr Peter Thomas

This comprehensive and practical book covers the complete range of allergies and sensitivities, from diet to environment. It tells you clearly and simply what to do to avoid allergies and how to deal with them when they arise. To be published shortly.

High blood pressure at your fingertips
Dr Julian Tudor Hart, with a chapter on pregnancy by Dr Wendy Savage

Julian Tudor Hart uses all his 26 years of experience as a General Practitioner and expert on blood pressure to answer your questions on high blood pressure. This book has been approved by the British Heart Foundation. To be published shortly.

Diabetes at your fingertips
NEW THIRD EDITION
Professor Peter Sönksen, Dr Charles Fox and Sister Sue Judd

461 questions on diabetes are answered clearly and accurately.

> ". . . you'll find this book a big help."
> *Gary Mabbutt,*
> *England International Footballer*

Parkinson's at your fingertips
Dr Marie Oxtoby and Professor Adrian Williams

Full of practical help and advice for people with Parkinson's disease and their families. This book gives you the information and the confidence to tackle the challenges that PD presents and to live a full, active life.

> '. . . I have learned a good deal . . .'
> *L. Buckley, Hants*

Epilepsy at your fingertips
Brian Chappell and Dr Richard Appleton

If you are one of the 420,000 people in the UK with epilepsy, you will find this practical book invaluable. It covers all the questions you will want to ask to allow you to manage the condition and achieve control of your life. Topics covered include: diagnosis; treatment; education; work; living with epilepsy; leisure; the future. To be published shortly.

PRIORITY ORDER FORM

Cut out or photocopy this form and send it (post free in the UK) to:

Class Publishing Customer Service
FREEPOST (no stamp needed)
LONDON W6 7BR

Tel: 01752 695745

Fax: 01752 695668

Please send me urgently
(tick boxes below)

**Post included
price per copy
(UK only)**

☐	**Asthma at your fingertips**	£14.95
☐	**Allergies at your fingertips**	£14.95
☐	**High blood pressure at your fingertips**	£14.95
☐	**Diabetes at your fingertips**	£14.95
☐	**Cancer information at your fingertips**	£14.95
☐	**Parkinson's at your fingertips**	£14.95
☐	**Epilepsy at your fingertips**	£14.95

TOTAL: _____

Easy ways to pay
Cheque: I enclose a cheque payable to Class Publishing for £_____
Credit card: please debit my ☐ Access ☐ Visa ☐ Amex ☐ Switch

Number: _____ Expiry date: _____

My address for delivery is

Name _____

Address _____

_____

Town _____ County _____ Postcode _____

Telephone number (in case of query) _____

Class Publishing's guarantee: remember that if, for any reason, you are not satisfied with these books, we will refund all your money, without any questions asked. Prices and VAT rates may be altered for reasons beyond our control.